The Group System

The Therapeutic Activity Group in Occupational Therapy

Barbara Borg, MA, OTR

Mary Ann G. Bruce, MS, OTR

SLACK Incorporated, 6900 Grove Road, Thorofare, New Jersey 08086

Managing Editor: Amy E. Drummond
Publisher: John H. Bond

Printed in the United States

Library of Congress Catalog Card Number: 89-043517

ISBN: 1-55642-065-X

Published by: SLACK Incorporated
                6900 Grove Road
                Thorofare, NJ 08086-9447

Last digit is print number: 10 9 8 7 6 5 4

Dedicated to Andrew, Emily,
Juan Carlos, John
and our parents

Contents

List of Figures

About the Authors

Barbara Borg and Mary Ann G. Bruce have been friends and colleagues since 1970. They have shared clinical and academic views, held similar positions in occupational therapy practice and education, and more recently, collaborated on numerous scholarly projects. They co-authored *Frames of Reference in Psychosocial Occupational Therapy* published by Slack, Inc., in 1987. This current text is the result of their interests in system theory, the relationship between theory and practice in group treatment and their continued excitement about the effectiveness of therapeutic activity groups in occupational therapy.

Barbara Borg graduated from Colorado State University with a bachelor of science degree in occupational therapy, and from the University of Northern Colorado with a master of arts degree in agency counseling. After working in adolescent and adult psychiatry as a staff occupational therapist and administrator, she worked in a private agency doing individual, couple, and family counseling. For several years she taught as an assistant professor in the Department of Occupational Therapy at Colorado State University, Fort Collins, Colorado. Currently Ms. Borg divides her professional time between writing and private practice.

Mary Ann Bruce holds a bachelor of science in occupational therapy from Colorado State University and a masters in counseling from Southern Connecticut State University. She has been an associate professor and department chairman at Quinnipiac College, Hamden, Connecticut and an associate professor and interim program director at the University of Texas Health Science Center, San Antonio. Currently she is in private practice and pursuing a doctoral degree in cognition and human development.

Introduction

A group context for treatment appreciates and makes use of the need all persons have on one hand to be themselves as individuals; while on the other hand to reach beyond themselves and relate to others in groups. Starting with their family, each person's involvement in groups at play, at school, at work and in the community develops throughout his or her life. In a sense, we are all experts, since each of us has had years of first-hand experience. However, when students or practicing therapists function as group leaders, they frequently need to bring all that they have learned into clearer focus.

In this book we discuss the small, therapeutic group. Our intent is to help the reader integrate what he or she has already learned about groups from personal experience with what each has gained through professional reading, and to then apply this to the activity group experience.

Occupational therapists who are interested in using therapeutic activity groups in either physical rehabilitation or in mental health settings, are faced with a problem: they often must extrapolate information from literature of group psychotherapy, which is primarily an analytic, verbal process, or from literature of sociology and communication theory, whose groups are highly task-oriented, but not involved in therapy. When talking about small, therapeutic activity groups, we emphasize that although they share some features in common with these other group models, they are unique in their own way right.

The whole is more than the sum of its parts. Kurt Lewin (1951) and von Bertalanffy (1969) relied heavily on this cornerstone of system theory; both provided much of the theoretical foundation for this book. We hold that, what is encountered in any group must be conceived as not only its elements and transactions in isolation, but something beyond; thus the group leader who is trying to integrate diverse information about the activity group needs a means to think about this greater whole. A system perspective is one such means, and it is the one we, as well as others, selected and developed in this discussion. We were attracted to system theory not only for its theoretical plausibility, but for the ease with which it could be practically applied to the discussion of small, therapeutic activity groups. The system perspective, with its emphasis on the wholeness of the group experience, acts as an organizer that can help the student and clinician select from information and derive meaning in order to make daily clinical decisions. The need for us as group leaders to make sense of our experience and to "think on our feet" is not likely to diminish, even in the ever-changing landscape of the therapeutic milieu.

One of the things we emphatically have wanted to avoid in our material is the suggestion that therapists discard their current theories in order to become system theorists. As the concept is developed within this text, a system-oriented approach accomodates the beliefs of a wide number of sound theory and practice models.

Trained and experienced as occupational therapists and counseling therapists, we hold a firm belief in the unique opportunity for growth available within therapeutic activity groups. But, we don't find that trying to force a task group or verbal psychotherapy group model onto the activity group is the best way to realize this potential. For that reason, we have tried to draw attention to what is unique to the therapeutic activity group.

We have observed that many current occupational therapy groups are moving away from the use of a verbal review of the activity group, a function we refer to as "processing the activity." Although not every activity can or needs to be processed, we have paid special attention to this group aspect, because we feel this can help patients integrate and profit from their group experience.

A major goal on our presentation of the material in this book has been to provide practical information to group leaders, often through the use of examples. We also want the reader to be drawn into the process of enactive learning, and have, therefore, posed many questions to be considered by the reader who must ultimately assimilate and apply the material.

As an additional resource, we conclude by summarizing a number of therapeutic activity groups that have been discussed in the literature, or are otherwise familiar to us. In some instances, we have personal experience with the groups presented, but we have chosen to use the references cited so that the interested reader might explore the literature further.

The groups selected are a fairly representative sample of the kinds of activity groups, currently conducted, especially in their diversity. Second, although there is more information available regarding some groups than others, we feel that there is enough information that the therapist could model a group after the ones described. Third, most of the groups described could be modified or structured to meet the needs of various patient populations.

Finally, we hope that these group summaries will illustrate vividly how the varying elements of the group can and do come together to create a therapeutic experience that can not be adequately understood by looking at any single element, but only as a reflection of the greater whole.

PART I

1
The Therapeutic Activity Group

Focus Questions

1. What is a small therapeutic activity group?
2. By what means can one synthesize and organize what is known about groups, therapy, and activity?
3. What is general system behavior theory?
4. What is a system model?
5. How is general systems theory applied to group treatment?
6. What are the relevant components in a therapeutic activity group?

Defining Therapy

There are several key concepts that influence any discussion of therapy activity groups. At its heart, this book is concerned with the art and science of therapy. Just what is "therapy"? What are therapists trying to do when they strive to make an activity therapeutic?

In health care, *therapy* refers to a formalized process, a contract between care-giver and patient. The client or patient is at the center of the therapy process. That is, the patient (if at all possible) makes known his or her needs and expectations for the therapeutic experience. The therapist makes a commitment to use knowledge and skills vis-a-vis acceptable methodologies to help the patient achieve those goals that are mutually agreed upon. Thus, therapy, as the term is commonly used, includes an organized system of data gathering, assessment, goal setting, treatment planning, treatment implementation, process review, documentation, as well as a means to ensure equality and enable accountability.

As was discussed in a previous publication (Bruce and Borg 1987), patient "needs" usually suggest that some kind of change is necessary. People change throughout their lives, and change can be regarded as an opportunity to improve one's quality of life. The patients seen in treatment may want to make specific changes in how they feel about themselves or their experiences. They may need a change in knowledge, either by acquiring new information or by experimenting with a new way of putting information together. They may need a tangible change in skill or behavior. An important adjunct to this idea of change is that persons involved in therapy experiences are unable to make necessary changes on their own—they require assistance. The anticipation of change can be both enticing and scary. Helpers are reminded that making desired changes can be difficult for patients, change may not easily occur, and the desire for change must exist within the individual.

The Group: A Relationship System

In mental health and physical medicine, one of the identified media of change is the group experience. As used in this book, a *treatment group* can be thought of as the intentional bringing together of individuals into a system of relationships in order to enable the satisfaction of member needs. In his introductory remarks for his book *Inpatient Group Psychotherapy,* Irving Yalom (1983, 5) provides a startling run-down of the diverse groups he encountered when visiting inpatient psychiatric programs across the country. As he states:

> The range of groups offered on the wards I visited was astonishingly broad (even allowing for the fact that similar groups may be named differently on different wards) and includes: interactional groups, analytic groups, multifamily groups, goals groups, movement therapy groups, art therapy groups, massage therapy groups, transition groups, relaxation groups, guided fantasy groups, dance therapy groups, music therapy groups, horticulture group therapy, medication education groups, future-planning groups, therapeutic community groups, living skills groups, craft groups, human sexuality groups, discharge-planning groups, problem-solving groups, rap groups, awareness-training groups, motor skills groups, assertiveness training groups, behavioral effectiveness groups, focus groups, Ann Landers groups, psychodrama groups, men's groups, women's groups, structured exercise groups, family-living groups, decision-making groups, puppetry groups, emotional identification groups, soap-opera discussion groups, task (project) groups, activity groups.

Common Group Characteristics

Like the groups outside of the treatment community, these treatment groups share some common characteristics. Members see themselves as a "group". They share some norms, values, and goals, and there is an inter-dependence among group members. In order for the group to truly experience itself as a group, there must also be a group process of inter-actions. Something must happen in the form of an exchange of ideas, influence, or action. The extent to which group feeling is experienced can be influenced by the frequency of contact. Groups with a "short life" may have participants who feel less ownership and are less aware of common characteristics.

An important focus in the understanding of group experiences is that of group process, also referred to as group dynamics.

Group Process

Current knowledge of group process has come through many chan-nels. The group experience has been studied from virtually every conceiv-able avenue, including anthropology, sociology, psychiatry, psychology, ecology, technology, even mathematics. Treatment or therapy groups have a history in the sociometric work of Moreno in the 1920s (Endnote #1), the therapeutic community of Maxwell Jones in Great Britain in the 1940s (Endnote #2), in the activity-group therapy developed by Slavson and others in the 1930s for use with children (Endnote #3), the Freudian or analytically based adult therapy groups (Endnote #4), and the encounter group movement of the 1960s and 1970s (Endnote #5). While the 1950s saw a popularization of analytic one-to-one therapy, group treatment had a resurgence in the 1960s with advances in the use of medications to treat mental illness. Medications enabled the deinstitutionalization of many chronically disturbed individuals and their subsequent treatment in community mental health settings.

The understanding of group process was advanced in nontherapy groups by the work of Kurt Lewin and those involved in the National Training Laboratories. This organization, under the auspices of the National Education Association, facilitated group experiences designed to teach group process to educators. Training groups, or T-groups, as they were called, came to be frequently used by industry as a means to teach group principles to management personnel, and to increase awareness of interpersonal relationships, and emotional factors (de Mare and Kreeger 1974; Verny 1974).

Work in the fields of anthropology and paleontology has contributed to the fund of knowledge that exists about groups. However, it is important to remember that while there are many common features among the groups studied in these and related fields, the studies obtained in one area do not necessarily translate to conclusions to be drawn in another. As a practical illustration, it is evident that a group of Boy or Girl Scouts does not function identically to a group of teamsters, business executives, or borderline patients. Yet, if one looks carefully at any small functioning group, it becomes apparent that a group is more than the simple sum of its parts. Treating eight patients individually for one hour each day is not the same as seeing them together in a one-hour treatment group. Understanding how a group takes on its own identity and influences its members is key to appreciating the means by which group treatment experiences can be so potent.

The Activity Group

The focus for this book is the activity group, special kind of therapeutic group used in occupational therapy. Many authors (Yalom 1970, 1983; de Mare and Kreeger 1974; Greenberg-Edelstein 1986; Duncombe and Howe, 1985) have distinguished between a group that is primarily verbal psychotherapy in orientation and one that is primarily task related. Most, however, acknowledge that there often exists some blurring in function: task groups can be therapeutic and verbal therapy groups can have some task-orientation.

In verbal psychotherapy, member interaction is supported to resolve interpersonal issues among members. The primary emphasis is on group *process*, and verbal interaction is the primary means of interaction.

In a task group, interaction is encouraged so that the group might accomplish an identified task (e.g., to solve a group problem) or provide a service.

The emphasis in the task group is the achievement of an identified *end product:* either specific decisions, recommendations or tangible results. Task groups have been identified in the literature of occupational therapy (Mosey 1981; Fidler 1969, Howe and Schwartzburg 1986) and have been studied extensively by sociologists who are interested in the ability of small task groups in business, the community, etc., to get a job done.

De Mare and Kreeger (1974) in Great Britian identify a therapeutic activity group in a way consistent with our own observations and experiences in the United States mental health system. They see therapeutic activity groups such as those carried out by occupational, recreational, art, poetry, music, and movement therapists and others using action techniques as part of their group as representing a process that is somewhere between verbal psychotherapy and a task group. In an activity group, interaction can be toward a shared group goal, as in task groups, but member interaction is considered as important as the larger goal. Verbal interaction is often an important part of the activity group, but just as often, interaction may be through the medium of the activity itself.

To illustrate: An occupational therapy group might involve a group of patients cooperating to prepare and serve a meal. In this case, the end product (the meal) is important, but so is the process of socialization that occurs among the patient group. Another group might have several patients listening together to a Tchaikovsky symphony or some hard-rock music. Members might be asked to share their reactions verbally or asked to share in a nonverbal way by creating their own music on some available musical instruments. In this second group, there may be no specific end product, and the process of communicating (verbally or musically) is the goal. A different activity group could be task-oriented, e.g., when a group of patients get together to repaint the dayroom, or paint a mural. However, unlike a task-group one might find in business, a therapeutic activity group considers the opportunity for social interaction, social learning, changes in member feelings, and life enrichment for each participant as important as the group's collective effect on the environment.

Another kind of activity group that is neither solely product nor process oriented is one in which patient education is the primary purpose. Education has a major role in groups providing support and knowledge to manage chronic diseases (e.g., arthritis and diabetes). During these support groups, patients learn about the disease process and medical management of symptoms, get advice regarding problems related to the chronic illness, and gain support from group members as they share experiences and attempt problem-solving.

Group Continuum and Activity Selection

How the activity is used to achieve the goals established for group members and what specific activities or tasks will be selected depends on the nature of the participants, the goals of treatment, the theoretical beliefs of the therapist (or how he or she feels goals can best be achieved), and many other elements discussed in the remainder of this text. Here we suggest a continuum for understanding the focus of the group, with psychotherapy groups tending to be the most process oriented, task groups least, and activity groups having a flexibility to use both a product and process orientation, and both verbal and nonverbal media. This continuum does *not* suggest that any of these three major types of groups need to be all or nothing in terms of process or product, verbal or activity media. For instance, it has become quite common for psychotherapists to use activities as a way to facilitate member interaction in a "warm up." Also, an activity group may involve member interaction around "interpersonal issues" in specific instances. It becomes a matter of looking at the group's emphasis and primary mission. Figure 1.1 depicts a group continuum that suggests the group's emphasis for treatment.

Psychotherapy Groups	Therapeutic Activity Groups	Traditional Task Groups
Goals: To provide a corrective emotional experience To resolve inter and intra- personal emotional issues	Goals: To build social skills To enable change in member feeling, thought, or skill	Goals: To accomplish a specified group task
Process emphasis	Product and process emphasis	Product emphasis (Outcome can be physical or cognitive)
Verbalization is primary medium	Verbalization and activity are primary media	Task is primary medium
Cooperation not emphasized apart from member needs	Cooperation may or may not be emphasized	Cooperation emphasized
Group needs can't be understood apart from member needs	Group and member needs both emphasized	Member needs often put aside for the good of the group (to enable task accomplishment)
Leader selects participants	Leader may or may not select participants	Leader may or may not select participants
Therapy is goal	Therapy is goal	Therapy need not be goal

Figure 1.1 Group Continuum

Group Size

What is a small group, as opposed to a large group? When the term "small" is used the reader may substitute the term "optimum size." Studies suggest that for a group to be most effective as a medium of change, it has to be large enough to allow for an adequate exchange of ideas, yet not be so large that participants can 'get lost' within the group (Tubbs 1984, Yalom 1983, de Mare and Kreeger 1974, Fisher 1980). From five to ten participants has been suggested as an ideal working number. For practical reasons, therapeutic activity groups may be larger than ten at times, or the number may dip below five. Larger groups may end up subdividing into smaller cliques in order for members to achieve the kind of interaction they seek; smaller groups may find themselves short on energy and/or resources. However, there are no specific rules.

There may be a treatment setting with a group composed of many patients working on their own projects or doing an individualized exercise program under the supervision of the therapist. This has been likened to the parallel play of young children (Mosey 1973). This is certainly a "group of patients" and may be a necessary experience for patients learning to become comfortable in groups. However this does not fit the kind of activity group described in this book. Group interaction in these cases is not being emphasized as a means of change.

Chapter Summary

In this chapter we have discussed the characteristics that help define the small therapeutic activity group. With so many groups being conducted within and outside of therapeutic settings, we feel it important to provide clear boundaries as regards the scope of this book.

As a means to compare our and the reader's understanding, we ask you, the reader, to do the following activity. As authors, we share our reactions in Endnote 6.

Reader Activity

Which, if any, of these group experiences do you think is a bonafide small therapeutic activity group, as it has been presented?

(a) Alana, Burt and Char are adult in-patients at a private psychiatric setting. One Saturday afternoon they had a block of unscheduled time. Because all three had full privileges (could leave the hospital with permission), they asked to go together to a local mall to browse and perhaps have a cup of coffee. The staff on duty felt good about the initiative the three had taken in finding a way to occupy their own time, and felt that the social contact among them would be beneficial. The staff gave them the go-ahead, but did ask that the three patients report in upon their return. After the patients returned to the institution, a staff member sat down with each of them briefly to discuss the outing. The outing was noted in each patient's chart.

(b) The patients receiving treatment at Johnstown Community Mental Health Center often move to a halfway house nearby, as an interim step towards independent living. They continue, while at the halfway house, to meet with a primary therapist, usually a social worker or counselor from the Mental Health Center. At the halfway house, two staff members from the Community Health Center meet with the residents on a biweekly basis in a group to help residents manage the practical issues of living together. At their last meeting, the group planned an outdoor barbecue to be carried out by and for the residents.

(c) The eight patients in a prevocational group at the McPhearson Rehabilitation Institute are preparing for re-entry into the community and attend an employment preparation group three times a week. During one of the sessions, the patients are given a resume format and asked to write a personal resume. Following the completion of a rough draft, during a group discussion clients share a summary of their employment history and state their work strengths and one area in which they need to change their work habits. The intent of the group is to produce a resume that can be used in the client's job search and to provide opportunities for group members to practice sharing verbally their employment history (as one does during an interview).

(See Endnote 6 for the authors' view).

Group in a System Model

Focus Questions
1. What is a system?
2. What are the system's component parts?
3. How does a system function?
4. What is the role of feedback?
5. What are the elements in the activity group system?

A group can be viewed as a system of relationships. It is a system with integrated elements such as those previously introduced (therapy, small group milieu and activity experience). To understand the integrated relationships within groups, we have selected a system model. System models and theories are not new but are becoming more prevelant in descriptions of group process and health care delivery. (Brill, 1985, Fisher 1980, Glick et al. 1987, Hoffman 1981, Liff 1979, Gruen 1979, Miller and Miller 1981). Before proceeding, we pause and qualify the meaning of the term *system theory* as is used in this text.

Definition of the System

A *system* is an organized entity of interdependent component parts. As the name implies, *system theory* is a way to think about how a system works. You may have come across system discussions in relation to technology (e.g., computers and "systems analysis") or in the physical, biologic, and social sciences (e.g., the nervous system, the family system). Although the meaning of system is not identical in all these diverse fields, parallel developments and terminology exist.

The simplest system in technology is often illustrated by the feedback loop (Fig. 2.1).

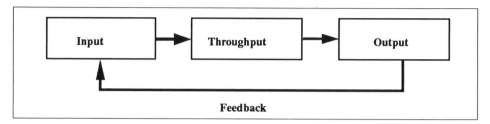

Figure 2.1   System Model (Closed System)

The feedback loop is a four part conceptual model of input, through-put, output and feedback. Anyone with access to a computer probably understands the meaning of this model:

1. Energy in the form of information comes into the computer. This is *input.*

2. The computer transforms or processes the information. This is the process of *throughput.*

3. Once the information has been transformed, the computer displays it on the screen as *output.*

4. The computer then stores this information and integrates it into what it already holds. This information becomes information for future transactions. This final function is accomplished by means of a feedback loop, or just *feedback.*

This scheme has promoted the analogy of person to machine and is used to depict human function in the works of Heinz Werner (1948, 1957), Allen Newell and Herbert Simon (1972), and others. It is, however, limited in its usefulness, in part because it doesn't convey the level of complexity, spontaneity, willfulness, and adaptation of which the person is capable.

General System Theory

Biologist Ludwig von Bertalanffy proposed a more encompassing system theory that pertained particularly to living systems, but also spoke of the relationship of the infinite numbers and kinds of systems. This he termed *general system theory.* (von Bertalanffy 1968) (Endnote #7). He saw systems as composed of *component parts* and also of component *relationships.* One can think of the parts of the system as juxtaposing with each other to make up the system's *structure.* The activity in the system is called the system's *function.* For example, a baseball team is composed of individual ball players (the 'parts'), who play assigned positions in a certain way—this creates the team's structure. The function of the team (playing ball) can only be understood by looking at how the 'parts' play together, or how they behave in relation to each other.

Keeping with this analogy, the way to understand the living system (here, a team) is to consider how all the parts or players work together. Any play made by any player affects the whole team. As stated by von Bertalanffy, we need to recognize that all parts of a living system interact with all the other parts, and that the only way to appreciate the richness of the system is to view it as a 'whole', and not in terms of individual parts, or a series of discrete relationships.

To distinguish living systems from machines, von Bertalanffy termed the former *open systems*. As open systems, living organisms possess energy which they use in their constant interaction with their environment. They are capable of seeking out what they need and taking it from the environment, and they are able to become more complex. Put another way, living organisms can change themselves when necessary. This is *not* possible, of course, in the machine. Not only did von Bertalanffy look at the relationships within an identified system, he recognized that systems are a part of and interact with greater systems. For example, the cell (a system within itself) exists within the nervous system, which is part of the person system, who lives within the family system which functions as part of the community, and so on. If there is a change in the nervous system of a person (for example, he or she is injured in a car accident), the whole person is affected. The individual's family will be affected as well as his or her contributions to the community. If, conversely, there is a change in a person's community (for example, a major corporation decides to move) the individual's own job security may be affected, may cause stress within the family, which may result in actual physiologic change within the individual's nervous system. This simplified example illustrates that, in the system perspective, all parts of the interacting systems are interdependent in relation to all other parts, and thus the whole context in which the system functions is important.

Personality as a System

Much of what von Bertalanffy wrote pertained to the person in particular. Von Bertalanffy considered general system theory as a framework that could be used to understand and describe personality, and he proposed that it was far more suitable than any of the frameworks that were most prevelent, as for example, analytic and behavioral theories (von Bertalanffy 1968,107-8, 205-18).

While not everyone agrees that practitioners and group leaders need to substitute general system theory for other frames of reference, general system theory does provide an over-arching structure that works well when using one of the many possible theoretical frameworks in a group setting. Summarized here are the most salient features of the general system view of personality. The three features of personality emphasized are those related to the person's ability to function in a group: the ability to (1) be *active* (2) be *organized* and (3) use an effective system of *boundarying*. Influencing these three functions, and in a sense an integral part of them, is the personality's ability to use or adapt to the consequences of the behavior it has produced through the successful incorporation of feedback.

An Active Person

The person is first and foremost a 'system' that must be conceived as an integrated whole. The person as an open system has the ability to take what he or she needs from the environment. This implies the ability and, in fact, the necessity to be active. People are action or 'doing' oriented. Their activity involves a give and take of energy within the environment. One of the things occupational therapists look at carefully in activity groups is the extent to which individual group members actively participate in the group experience. This can be thought of as their ability to mobilize personal energy. Anyone who has worked with patients in groups realizes that not every patient wants to be active in the group or in his or her own life experiences. The ability to be active is influenced by (a) the person's level of energy, (b) the present state of motivation, (c) the degree to which he or she feels competent to initiate and pursue what he or she needs, and (d) the extent to which the individual feels the group experience provides something that he or she wants. Von Bertalanffy proposed that the motivation for activity comes from within the person and is experienced as the need to create and find new and challenging experiences. Tapping into this inner drive is consistent with the goals of some of the activity groups that will be described in this text. However, general system theory acknowledges that finding new challenges is predicated on a base of safety and the meeting of essential physical and emotional needs. Maslow's often-cited hierarachy of needs (Endnote #8) is, therefore, consistent with general system theory's view of personhood. We recognize that not all patients come into treatment with a healthy 'activating' system, nor are basic safety and psycho-physical needs already met. Therefore, the therapist selects and structures a group activity to reflect this understanding.

An Organized Person

Also implied in von Bertalanffy's work and discussed in more detail by Liff (1979) is that a sound personality system (the healthy person) is well *organized*; that is, the various systems and sub-systems work well together to meet the person's needs.   One can conceive of both internal and external organizations.   When persons are *internally* organized, they are able to make sense of experiences and put them into a meaningful mental context.   When they are *externally* organized, they can then act upon what they know and respond in a way that, too, is organized, that has a pattern and that fits with what others are doing and expect from them. In practice, the patients that are extremely disorganized are often those who get the psychiatric label of psychosis. One of the things that health care professionals have learned is that organizing the environment and giving very clear messages to the disorganized person can help with his or her reorganizing process. Thus, when occupational therapists structure the group activity, they pay particular attention to the demands it makes for member organization and the extent to which it can help organize the group experience for specific participants.

Personal Boundaries

Related to both the ability to be both active and organized is the individual's ability for effective *boundarying*. We can recall that von Bertalanffy distinguished between closed and open systems. The person, he said, functions as an open system. Clearly, however, not everyone is equally open in their give-and-take with the environment. You have probably heard one person describe another as being "closed," referring to the other's refusal to consider new experiences or relationships. This person can be viewed as having overdeveloped boundaries, or may be described as "overdefended" (Liff 1979, 46). On the other hand, there are those who seem too nonselective, who believe everything they hear or take too much to heart; who don't discriminate wisely and try out experiences that are harmful. These persons have underdeveloped boundaries. *Boundaries* relate directly to the patient's ability to make use of group communication and feedback and the ability to try group activities.   Persons who have extremely dysfunctional boundarying systems may have unclear ideas about who they are and how they are separate from others.   Group experiences can be structured, and the environment can be used in such a way that those persons with tenuous boundaries are assisted in the boundarying process. Persons with impermeable or inflexible boundaries often have difficulty accepting feedback from group members or learning from an activity.

Personality as Part of Greater Systems

The discussion of personality thus far has focused on the function of personality (its ability to be active, organized and effectively boundaried). General system theory also emphasizes that personality must be seen in its greater social context if therapists are to understand how to make it easier for people to change or appreciate why effecting permanent change sometimes seems so difficult .

It has been characteristic of those in health care to focus on the individual and to pay lesser attention to changing the environment. This situation is understandable. It is the patient who is in treatment; it is with him or her that helpers contract. Additionally, all therapists have limitations in terms of what can be accomplished in a circumscribed time period. However, the therapist who recognizes the significance of the patient's home or anticipated enviroment will try to facilitate the acquisition of skills that enhance function in the patient's everyday world. This may include the therapist's helping patients identify where change must occur (either within themselves and/or in the environment) and what is inaccessible to change.

Summary of General System Theory

In summary, system theory attempts to describe how the component parts of an organized structure interact. General system theory, in particular, addresses open or living systems and stresses the need to view systems holistically within an environmental context. Although not sufficiently advanced in its development to be able to predict how components within a system will engage, general system theory is described by von Bertalanffy as a "guiding idea" that can be used in the social sciences to help make sense of human behavior. (von Bertalanffy 1968, 24).

The healthy functioning individual is characterized as one who is active, organized, and has effective but not overly stringent boundaries. The individual is motivated to act upon his or her environment and explore and master it, provided that the essential need for safety (emotional and physical) has been met. Like all activity, including that used in the maintenance of boundaries and organizational tasks, healthy function expends energy. In addition, the system assimilates new energy and new information through selectively permeable boundaries. As we discussed, these aspects of the person-as-a-system are given particular attention when therapists plan and lead therapeutic group activities.

System theory is not the first nor the only theoretical proposal that takes into account the importance of the environment, or that stresses the interrelationships within a structure. In many ways system theory is similar to gestalt and field psychologies such as that of Kurt Lewin (See Endnote #9), and brings to mind holistic models in medicine, as well as the human ecology studies of Urie Bronfenbrenner (1979) (See Endnote #10).

As stressed by Brill, system theory is a means to survey the human experience and put it into understandable context. For those in helping fields, its application can make it easier to identify where intervention is best carried out. (Brill 1985, 117).

A Group System Model

An open system approach has been applied to the study of small groups by Tubbs and, with some alteration, is the model used in this book. As Tubbs stresses, in order to understand small group interaction, one needs a way to manage a huge number of variables that affect the group experience. Tubbs states that he is attracted to the system model because it proposes a complex interrelationship of forces within the group. In other words, it "avoids the idea that complex behaviors in groups result from a single cause," (Tubbs 1984, 12). Although it is meant to show that groups function as open systems, Tubbs' model, as he depicts it schematically, is less than ideal because it resembles the simple feedback loop or the machine-like (closed) system to which von Bertalanffy and many others have objected.

In figure 2.2, Tubbs identifies three kinds of variables that roughly correspond to input, throughput, and output. The first set of variables (input) he calls *relevant background factors*, which are the attributes of the group participants. The second set of variables (throughput) he calls *internal influences*. These are the process components of the group—for instance, the way decisions are made, the style of leadership, the communication patterns, and the roles taken by individual group members.   The third set of variables (output) Tubbs calls the *consequences* of small group interaction. These consequences can include changes in participant's skills, thoughts, or feelings, and the 'solving' of a specified group problem or completion of a group task. The results or consequences of the group experience affect each member in some way (feedback), as well as the environment and the process of the group itself. Thus, Tubbs acknowledges that a change in any component of the group can affect change in relationship to any and all the other group components.

In summary, according to Tubbs *input* is the raw material of the group in the form of relevant background factors. *Throughput* refers to the internal group influences that occur in the course of the group activity. It comprises the processes of interaction and influences on these processes.

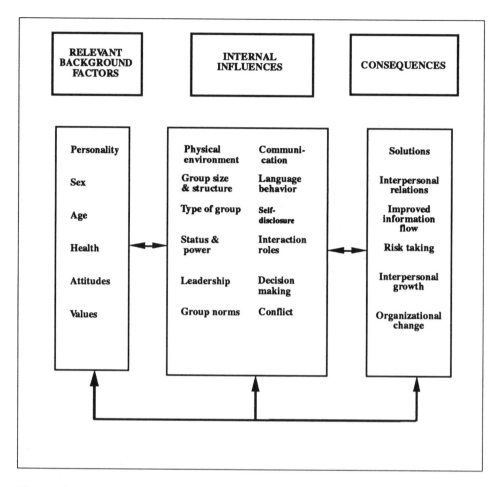

Figure 2.2 Open System Model. Reproduced with permission from S.L. Tubbs, A Systems Approach to Small Group Interaction, 2d ed., (New York: Random House, 1984), 43.

Output can be thought of as the end result or the outcome of the group interaction. However, beyond being merely an end, output provides new input for future interaction, and thus can be thought of as a "beginning." The process by which the consequences of group action are continually influencing members, group process, and future results is the cycle of *feedback.*

Tubbs' model is not specific to therapy groups and is concerned primarily with verbal interaction in verbally oriented groups. Using his model as a point of departure, we present a system model for activity group treatment (See Figure 2.3).

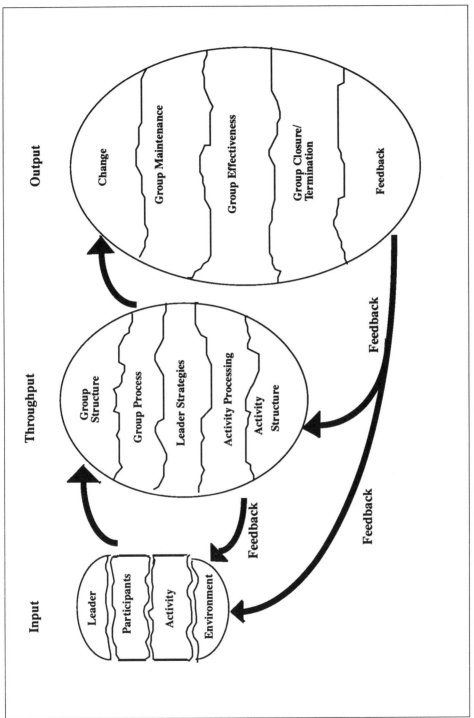

Figure 2.3   Therapeutic Activity Group as a System

Activity Group System

Input

As input or relevant background for the group we consider the following elements:

(a) treatment *environment,* which includes the specific physical attributes, time parameters, and "set". The environment is considered in   terms of what is valued and what is viewed as the mission of treatment.

(b) what the *participant* brings to the group, e.g., his or her strengths and limitations, preferred communication style, values, interests, perception about self as a group member, and personal goals. The therapist should pay particular attention to the extent the patient can participate and contribute in the group by considering his or her level of energy, ability to select information, maintain personal boundaries, and organize information and responses.

(c) the attributes of the *activity* around which the group is to be structured; e.g. creative, educational, skill, practice, etc.

(d) what the *therapist* brings into the group, including, for example, the therapist's area of expertise, limitations, preferred style, expectations, and level of energy. The theoretical beliefs, or "frames of reference" of the therapist and of the larger treatment setting will influence all aspects of input to the group.

When these four elements come together they interact and are influenced by the process known as throughput.

Throughput

The *throughput* of the group is the 'how and why' of the group's interaction. Throughput will also be influenced by the therapist's frame of reference, and may be reflected in the group's conception and construction according to a developmental model, an analytic model, a functional model, a motor-skills model, a cognitive/educational model, or other specified group framework. Throughput is most often described in terms of two dimensions.

(a) the *group's structure* includes the group's goals, therapeutic activity, organization (e.g., size, patient composition), and specific rules pertaining to how the group is run.

(b) the *group process* refers to the interactions that occur among the members (including the group leader), the manner in which group roles are assumed and fulfilled, the communication patterns in the group, and how the therapeutic activity is used and processed.

Outcome (Output)

The group *output or outcome* refers to a blending of individual change, group maintenance, feedback, and termination. Treatment outcomes include:

(a) changes that have come about within individual participants in thoughts, feelings, attitudes, and/or behaviors and

(b) changes made in the environment by the group as a whole. Treatment outcomes do not only result at the end of the activity, but may occur during its process.

The outcome also includes maintenance of the group. The interactions that occur during the group not only bring about individual change and produce an end product, they also identify, support, and further develop the group boundaries. The outcomes of all group interaction produce feedback.

As with Tubbs' and other system models, *feedback* exists as the constant interplay and influence of all parts of the system on all other parts. Feedback can go out into other systems, affecting individual growth and change. It also comes back into the system, influencing future activity groups.

Termination may also be an outcome of the activity group. When patients have participated in an open or closed activity group, and they have accomplished the group task or are being discharged from treatment, the group experience ends, and participants experience termination.

Chapter Summary

A system perspective can be used as an over-arching structure that helps one to manage and make sense of what contributes to the therapeutic activity group experience. As used in this book, a system view of groups is intended to complement and not replace those theories and beliefs about groups and therapy held by individual therapists. Given particular emphasis in the system model are the ability of the group as a whole and the ability of individual participants, to be effectively active, organized, and boundaried, to be open and responsive to the cycle of feedback, and to change in the direction of desired treatment outcomes.

3

Group Input: Environment and Patient Characteristics

Focus Questions:

1. How does the culture set expectations for what can or should occur in the group?

2. What is meant by the term "treatment milieu?"

3. How does the treatment milieu influence group goals, process and outcome?

4. What characteristics of the participants can be expected to influence the group?

5. What are the components of the patient system?

6. What in the environment influences group treatment?

The Environment

Think for a moment about what in the environment serves as a backdrop for the group experience. Keeping with a system approach one could look at the cultural environment, the community environment and the actual treatment setting. Because of limited space, this book touches only briefly on the larger socio-cultural and community environments, although it does not intend to minimize their importance.

The environment, in its most encompassing sense, includes the entire culture, its attitudes and beliefs about health, illness, health-care and nurturance, activity, dependence, independence, and all the attributes that contribute to these.

Despite the efforts made in health education, there is still discomfort in the populace over psychiatric and physical illness, and concerning differences and limitations. We cannot, in this text, explore these subjects, but the reader is probably aware of the real fears many people have of becoming ill or otherwise compromised in their ability to function. There is fear and discomfort, too, with being around others who are "different" or who have special problems.

Another fundamental cultural value that influences what occurs in groups (and helps determine who will participate in group treatment experiences)is related to nurturance. As discussed by Greenberg-Edelstein, nurturance is the root of group therapy and includes group actions of "aiding, comforting, confiding, nursing, exchanging . . .establishing solidarity and promoting development and growth." (Greenberg-Edelstein 1986, 1)

Every care-giver, every administrator, every third-party payer, and every patient and client brings with them a set of beliefs about health, illness, and caring and activity based on the physical, social, emotional, and economic realities that all share. To use a popular term, it is "awesome" to realize how much of what actually goes into and is expected from group treatment is shaped before any clinic or day-room door ever opens.

Treatment Milieu as a System

In most of the literature on group treatment, the environment addressed is the treatment setting, also called the treatment milieu. The milieu may be an inpatient or outpatient setting, may require patients to stay for a lengthy treatment period, or may serve as an evaluative placement center in which the population changes daily. The treatment milieu is also defined by the mission of the treatment program and/or institution, the specific care-givers involved in the therapy program and their roles, the treatment activities that are offered, and whether they are optional or mandatory. Milieus also influence the use of unstructured time, methods of decision making, and the chain of command. All of these components create a system that significantly influences the group experience, its possible accomplishments, and how it functions. As therapist-authors, we illustrate this milieu influence from our own experience.

Culture Supports Group Treatment

Several years ago, we worked as occupational therapists at a psychiatric facility with two treatment arms: one a privately funded in-patient, acute care setting, and the other an out-patient facility that was directed towards acute, chronic, and after- care. At the time there was generally funding available from private insurance carriers and the federal government for lengthy psychiatric treatment. All treatment activities were considered part of the "therapeutic milieu" and were covered under one flat fee. The concept of the therapeutic community or therapeutic milieu conceived at this center was similar to that developed by Maxwell Jones (1953) Thus, all treatment activities plus all patient-staff interactions (both formalized and informal) were considered an opportunity for therapy and as valuable as one-to-one interaction between a patient and his or her admitting psychiatrist. The formalized group activities included those of psychodrama, occupational therapy, recreational therapy, family meetings, community meetings, and verbal group therapy. The message to the patient group, both implicit and explicit, was that treatment groups were valuable; that patient participation was expected; and equally important, that staff would support the patient's participation. Specifically, the staff would be there to be helpful if an individual was having difficulty with a particular treatment activity and to help patients to understand and integrate activity experiences.

The result, in most instances, was that patients came to therapy groups with a reasonably positive mind-set: they seldom asked to be excused from activities, and the therapist had the support of other treatment staff within a particular activity. Also, therapists usually knew how many patients to plan for in treatment groups, and seldom had to worry about the disruptive effects of patients being pulled from group activities.

The hospital 'mission' was to return patients as contributing members to the community and, when necessary, to provide after-care support. Seldom were patients admitted who were not considered to have rehabilitation potential, who were considered recalcitrant or chronically criminal. Because of its location in a rather affluent neighborhood and because of its religious sponsorship, many patients were from a middle to upper income group, and many had a Christian background. All these factors supported the treatment mission.

Laissez-Faire Attitude Toward Group Treatment

At another facility in the same city, also a privately funded psychiatric inpatient, acute-care setting, the hospital mission and population (in terms of demographics) were quite similar. However, at this institution the milieu was not considered as important as the private counsel between physician and patient. While occupational therapy and recreational therapy were also available, attendance was not required. Patients were told to attend if they wished. (See Endnote #11). Not surprisingly, many patients chose not to participate in activity based therapies, since the message conveyed was that these therapies were not important enough to be mandatory. The activity groups were provided by recreational and occupational therapists who expressed concern about the lack of support. Their morale was low. Many (but not all) patients only attended these milieu activities when they had "nothing else to do." Depressed patients usually lacked the motivation to attend at all. It is not that therapists lacked the neccessary skills. In fact, when therapists were able to interest individuals in attending therapy, often by means of striking up sound one to one alliances, some effective group activity therapy did evolve. However, by no means was the potential for these therapies met.

Contrasting Cultures Impact Group Treatment

A third type of setting frequently found in the mental health system is the psychiatric unit in a general hospital. In this setting, one may find a difference between the routines of the general hospital and those of a therapeutic milieu. Patients in these settings frequently have physical problems as well as psycho-social concerns. These physical symptoms may require a more traditional nursing approach, or call for treatments that interrupt the milieu group treatment schedule. Patients may have less energy to expend in groups because of physical illness or may assume that the benefits of hospitalization come from nursing care, medication, and rest (the traditional benefits identified with a stay in a general hospital), rather than investment and participation in the treatment groups (the benefits associated with treatment in milieu mental health settings). The function of ancillary services may also impact the milieu. For example, the hospital's kitchen usually provides individual trays so patients can eat in the privacy and comfort of their rooms. Traditionally, the therapeutic milieu supports patients' eating in a common dining room with ample opportunity for staff and patients to socialize during meals. Housekeeping services also have a different focus. Therapeutic milieus suggest that patients participate in maintaining their room environments; e.g., keeping their rooms orderly, making their bed daily, etc. General hospitals provide support staff who assume these responsibilities. Activities may also be viewed as "diversional" rather than as contributing to therapy and "wellness."

In some settings, the previously mentioned conflicts, as well as others, have been resolved, and the goals of the therapeutic community are achieved with some compromise. In other settings the conflict between treatment cultures provides the stimulus for interchange, staff education, and constant problem solving.

In these three contrasting examples, the set for activity group experiences is very different. They illustrate that both therapist and patient take from the treatment environment expectations about whether the group activity experiences will be successful and worth their time.

Additionally, not only does the treatment milieu provide a mental set for participation in groups, it acts as a source of information in terms of specific group functions and expectations. From interchanges with staff and patients, all in the treatment environment learn about expectations of group participants, actual group events, and the behavior tolerated or prohibited. The informal "chat" network may well be more influential in creating negative or positive expectations than any formalized explanation of group and treatment activities. It is not unusual, for example, to hear one patient tell another that at group meetings someone is "always wanting to know your feelings," or that at recreational therapy "you get to play and the staff lets their hair down," or that "at psychodrama people cry a lot."

The Inpatient and Outpatient Milieu

Dr. Yalom addressed at length the differences he perceived in an inpatient as opposed to an outpatient group milieu in psychiatry (Yalom 1983). That a fundamental difference exists is reiterated in the work of others (Corey 1978; Rice and Rutan 1987; Leopold 1977; Kaplan 1986). Although these authors are addressing group psychiatry, what they emphasize often becomes evident in physical care settings also.

Inpatient Milieu

In psychiatric treatment, as well as in physical medicine, inpatients are often in extreme distress and disorganization. The inpatient setting frequently provides acute care with the goal of managing symptoms and stabilizing patients, often by means of medications. The patient population is frequently very heterogeneous, with a wide span of age, social status, education, physical and psychiatric diagnoses; but a predominance of diagnoses indicative of severe dysfunction.

This type of setting might be typified by that found in a city or county hospital psychiatric wing. Individuals are often picked up and brought by the police because of their disruptive behavior in the community, or because they may be a threat to their own or the safety of others.

In such a setting, there may be a rapid turnover of patients. Groups that meet here often have to respond to the fact that patients have little time to be introduced and acclimatized to the group. Because patients may come in and out of a particular group situation quickly, it's often hard to establish a group feeling. Therapists may lack the opportunity to do an extensive evaluation to determine an individual's suitability for a particular group activity. Thus, the milieu is one of a quick-paced, often tumultuous arena in which staff respond to many crises. This will certainly influence group participants. Sometimes even those who are better organized are hard-pressed to maintain a sense of calm and find in their experiences a way to pursue their own therapy goals.

Outpatient Group

To draw an extreme contrast, one can look at the milieu of an outpatient group. As discussed by Yalom (1970, 1983), this is the group psychotherapy popularized by television and movies. Considered in its ideal, group members are selected by the therapist through a careful screening process to determine their suitability for the group. Many, but not all, consider it imperative to create a group population in which members have similar backgrounds, ages, and socio-economic levels. The participants are considered appropriate when they have the ability to be active, organized and effectively boundaried. The therapist believes that they will be able to contribute positively to an introspective dialogue, and that they will benefit from the experience. Such a group may contract to meet for an extended period of time (weeks, months to years), and once the group is filled, there may be little if any change in membership. The counterpart in physical medicine is represented by long-term groups in rehabilitation centers where individuals with diagnostically similar problems meet together for lengthy periods. The emotional and cognitive milieu of this group is often one of trust, optimism, expectation, and intensity.

The contrasting prototypes are just that: prototypes only. At some centers, for example, the inpatient activity groups may also be attended by day care and outpatients. In elderly and transitional living facilities, residents (inpatients) may have acute or chronic problems. Outpatient activity groups in the community are not necessarily the high-key groups of television either. Many are composed of those individuals needing continued support. The aftercare group in psychiatry, for instance, might be typified as having members, who are often marginally capable, with a tenuous commitment to therapy.

To summarize, Yalom's distinctions between in and outpatient groups are important because they have alerted helpers to the significance that such factors as length of patient stay, stability of group membership, patient composition, and overall milieu have on group process and group goals. These factors will influence group goals whether the groups are in physical medicine, psychiatry, or other health-care and community systems.

Physical Setting

One cannot consider the treatment milieu without assessing the physical setting in which group activity will occur.

At the first facility we previously described, there was a large, multi-room facility designated for occupational therapy. In many ways it represented the ideal. One room was minimally but comfortably furnished with living room furniture and wall-to-wall carpet. A homey atmosphere could easily be evoked and fit well with social oriented and daily living oriented activities.

A separate, utilitarian clinic with tile floors, easy-to-wipe counters, and movable tables and chairs provided a different setting that would encourage creativity with art media, exploration, and a sense of freedom to experiment. An enclosed patio further invited play and spontaneity and provided the feeling of being at one with nature.

Physical Boundaries

All of the rooms in this facility had several features in common. First, they had physical boundaries. The group could easily identify "This is where we meet," "This space is ours." Boundaries help a group to identify itself as a group and help minimize intrusion from nongroup members. If you need a reminder about how important physical space is to a group, try to remember back to when you were a child. Many of us can recall creating a club with a few special friends. Next to deciding who would be in and who out, the most important task seemed to be finding a place to meet, a special clubhouse. Often assembling the club "house" was a significant ritual, and its visibility served as proof that we were indeed a separate group.

Some early and very analytically oriented discussion of boundaries and physical space pertaining to group activities appears in the early works of Slavson (1950, 1961; Slavson and Schiffer 1975), and the interested reader might wish to explore these.

Physical boundaries help make real the emotional and cognitive boundaries that people experience. For those with limited ego strength and reality-testing, boundaries can help them to identify where they are and what is going on. Conversely, too much of a physical boundary can lead people to feel "cooped up." It is important that there be a clearly identified passageway from an enclosed space, plus, if possible, a window or skylight. Not every group activity experience can be arranged in its own room, nor is that always desirable. If the space for a group meeting is within a larger setting, the therapy experience can be set apart from the rest of the activities by means of portable screens, room dividers, or bookshelves. Even creating a circle with chairs or placing people in a circle establishes a sense of boundaries.

As was said, not all groups need strict bounds. Many groups meet in a less bounded setting that is 'natural' to the activity experience that is occurring. Cooking groups may meet in an area that simulates a normal kitchen, social groups in a living-room like space, and so on. Some group experiences are designed to take patients into the community. In these cases, group members often arrange to meet at restaurants, parks, and other public facilities; these group members do not need a consistent physical environment to know that they belong to the group, nor to get themselves to group meetings.

Some groups meet in environments designed to invite mobility, spontaneity, and interaction. By and large, in these groups therapists want patients to be able to move about and converse freely. Furniture is often lightweight and easily rearranged; supplies may *not* be under lock and key, and are within sight and reach so that group members might have access to them. (Exceptions will be made when patient protection and/or suicidal precautions are needed.)

This very flexible environment is not always appropriate. For example, if your group is striving to help members regain control or aiding in reinforcing reality, then you might want an environment where seating is not mobile and spontaneity not encouraged. If the group experience is built along the lines of a classroom or work experience, you also may want participation to be more formalized and commotion to be discouraged.

Other Kinds of Boundaries

The key is to recognize the environment's role as an organizing structure with specific boundaries. These boundaries can be conceived as physical, as well as containing cognitive-emotional messages about the kind of behavior that is expected. Borrowing from the traditional analytic model, many verbal group psychotherapists set up a physical environment that is devoid of ornaments. Simple seating and adequate lighting are all that are in the room where the group meets. The intent is to allow the group tone to be set by group members. However, activity group leaders are more likely to structure the environment in a way that promotes their particular activity. For example, using a round table with common work space and materials for collage making facilitates interaction and sharing during the work period and provides a more intimate space for the discussion that follows the completed collage.

Another important boundary is the time frame in which the group meets. Ongoing groups typically meet at a consistent time period. This consistency provides additional structuring information, e.g., "It's 9:00 A.M., I belong in my stress reduction group now."

Reader Activity

Before closing the discussion of the therapeutic environment, try to do the following exercise .

Suppose for a moment that you are about to be a group participant in a 35- minute poetry group. The group leader has copied the poem, "All I ever really needed to know I learned in Kindergarten" by Robert Fulghum, and each group member is given a copy. The poem will be read aloud, and the participants will be asked to share their reactions. Which of the following characteristics of the activity environment do you think would

1. Make you feel more comfortable?
2. Facilitate member interaction?
3. Be distracting?
4. Discourage member interaction?

• Bridge Over Troubled Waters playing softly in the background
• subdued lighting from table lamp; no other light source
• ceiling fluorescent lighting throughout room
• coffee pot plugged in and cups available at nearby counter
• aquarium with small fish on table next to group circle
• posters on wall, one with Teddy Bear, saying "I need a hug"
• patient art work scattered around room
• sound of telephone ringing at nurses' station, in the background
• unemptied ashtrays scattered around room
• large clock on wall behind leader's head
• floor cushions provide only seating
• folding chairs provide only seating

The Patient as a System

If one started listing all of the possible component systems or parts that exist within the person, one would not only be exhausted, one would lose a sense of the forest for the trees.

In her book, *Working with People*, Brill depicts the individual as composed of five major subsystems, each interacting to make up the greater person-system   (See fig. 3.1). Thinking of every individual as having a cognitive, physical, social, psychological, and spiritual self evokes the image of persons having many component 'parts' without losing the utility of a system   analogy.

Depending on the patient population and the therapeutic setting any of the preceding subsystems might be considered especially important when the group leader approaches the patient as a prospective group member. The therapist using activity groups in physical medicine, for example, might give greater relative emphasis to the physical system than the spiritual. The pastoral counselor might do the reverse. In a holistic systems approach, however, the need to pay some attention to all parts of the person in appreciating the whole is emphasized.

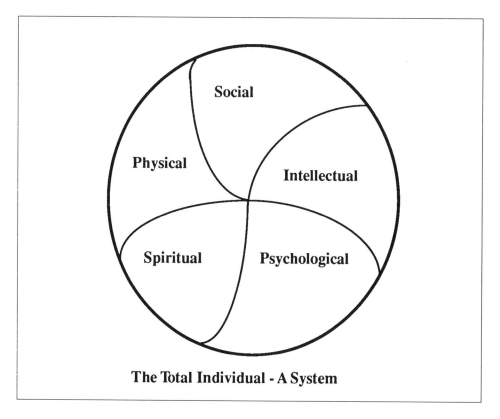

Figure 3.1   Person System

Patient Screening for Group Treatment

Because this book is intended to be a resource for therapists with varied treatment priorities who use more than one kind of activity group, we can't suggest a universal screening tool for selecting therapeutic activity group participants. However, in order to gain a general understanding of potential group members we propose that the therapist-leader address the following:

1. The patient's understanding of the reason for treatment.
2. The patient's strengths.
3. The patient's values.
4. The social situations which cause patient comfort or discomfort.
5. The patient's ability to be active, organized and effectively boundaried.

The Patient's Understanding
of Reason for Treatment

Not everyone comes into the treatment experience voluntarily or with a clear idea about the reasons for treatment. One of the first things therapists can do is help patients identify what has happened in their life that has resulted in their being in therapy. When confused, or just not well prepared for the therapy experience, the person may not be able to see self as the referent. The individual may say, "I'm here because my wife called the police and had me brought in." Or, "I'm here because my doctor thinks I need to be." Even when individuals place the burden squarely on themselves (e.g. "I'm here because I was afraid that I might kill myself"), they may not have a clear understanding of how the particular therapeutic experiences (here, the therapeutic activity group) can help them feel differently or "solve" their problems.

In an acute setting, therapists may have little opportunity to talk with prospective group members to assist them in orienting to the group experience. We've seen patients be checked into the hospital at 9:00 A.M. and be escorted by a staff member to a group activity at 10:00 A.M. This abrupt initiation to the group experience is not a fair beginning. We'd recommend that group leaders stay firm in their request that no one be brought into the group without some kind of orientation or preparation. (While not ideal, this could be done by a staff member other than the group leader who was familiar with the group's process, activities and goals. Some settings also have pamplets or other literature that outlines the treatment program and highlights the purpose of the therapeutic experiences.)

When patients do recognize that they have a need for change and see themselves as the central figure in the therapy process, they will often talk about themselves primarily in terms of their own failures and limitations. This can be true whether the limitations are physical, cognitive, social, emotional, or spiritual. For example, it is quite common for patients in psychiatry to have a history of unsuccessful group relationships, and this spills over into their expectations about themselves as activity group participants, influencing their skills. (Similarly, individuals dealing with physical changes may be focused on what they can no longer physically accomplish.)

The willingness to be an active group participant and commitment to the treatment process will be strongly influenced by their understanding of what they can hope to gain from the treatment experiences offered. At some point, each individual member needs to realize that the ultimate goal of participation is a change within him or her, while accepting the reality of limitations that may exist. Even if the environment proves to be a barrier, the patient needs to find a better way to cope with it, and a means to change his or her relationship to it.

If a patient has no apparent idea of what he or she needs to do in treatment, nor how a group experience can be helpful, it is not realistic to expect that everything will be accomplished before or during the first group meeting. Therapists can use their initial contacts with patients to give simple explanations introducing them to the group experience. For example, we might say "It sounds like you've had difficulty feeling that there's anything worthwhile you can do. I want you to participate in the group because I believe it will give you the chance to relate to people in a way that is different from what you've been experiencing." Or, "I hope you'll have a chance to be with people in a more playful way, one that will be a lot less stressful than the way you've had to relate at work." Or, "I'm placing you in a group with people who have similar physical limitations, who need to increase their endurance as you do. I think you'll find that the group can be a source of support for all of you."

The Patient's Strengths

Therapists are not only or even mostly concerned with the patient's limitations. There are all kinds of strengths, some which can be identified with a particular sub-system (e.g., "I'm strong. I like that I have a lot of physical endurance."); others which address how human subsystems work together as a whole (e.g., "I feel that I am a pretty good mother"). It can be very difficult for people in treatment to relate to their strengths or things that they like about themselves. Sometimes when the therapist asks patients to identify positive things about themselves, they respond something like the child that has been scolded, "I'm bad; there's nothing I can do right anymore," or, "Everyone is disappointed with me." Older adults sometimes respond in a way that suggests that their value lay in the past; for example, "I used to be good at ... , but now I'm useless."

Often times, therapists become aware of their patients' strengths, not from anything patients have said, but from their observations of and interactions with them. One way that helpers can introduce the idea of 'positives' is to share aloud their discovery; e.g., "Terry, I enjoyed your song! I had no idea that you enjoyed performing. Your voice is lovely!" or, "Thanks for helping with the equipment, Mark. That was really kind and helpful of you."

One of the most interesting things that has become apparent over the years in which we have worked with patients and students, and in our own lives, is the realization that one's strengths are often just a margin beyond one's weaknesses. For example, the person who is so emotional that every comment seems to hurt his or her feelings, may also be the person who is sensitive and responsive to the needs of others. The child who is stubborn at school may, in a positive sense, have the strength of his or her convictions when it comes to standing up for important ideals. Thus, it can be helpful to point out the relationship of what one normally thinks of as positive and negative attributes, especially when working with patients, to help keep them from disowning what they see as 'bad' about themselves.

Also remember that both human strengths and limitations are lived out within specific environmental (internal and external) boundaries. For instance, I am probably not always a good listener or hard worker; conversely, I am not always late, nor unable to "do anything with my hands." Rather, I may be a patient listener with my colleagues at work, and only so-so when the newsboy is trying to sell me on the local paper. Or, I might not be proficient at what people consider crafts, but I do a good job of repairing things around the house.

During group experiences, through the structure and process of the activity, therapists enable patients to feel or see the strengths they have and encourage patients to build upon their strengths, while becoming more accepting of themselves as "whole" people.

The Patient's Values

Ask young children what is most important to them and they might answer, "my bike" or "toys" without hesitation. Ask adults, and they may have to think much longer to select from a number of answers. Among the things people value are possessions, ideas, relationships, accomplishments and time. What anyone values is inexorably tied up with their own life experiences and their identity. There are a couple of generalizations that can be made regarding values. First, few people want to be involved in an experience that they feel has little value or purpose. Second, if someone is going to be an active participant in a therapy experience, that person needs to feel that it relates to his or her values.

It is easy at times for therapists to get caught up in the values common to therapy. For instance, helpers tend to value behavior that is appropriately assertive, that is open, and that pertains to feelings. But, what do patients value? Assertiveness, for instance, may seem rude, even a disgrace, to those persons with Mexican-American or Oriental roots. The older adult may have a value system in which it is discourteous to say negative things about others, or to bring the spotlight of attention to oneself. Values are personal; they are also a reflection of the families in which people are raised, their schools, the communities they hailed from, and their places of worship. From a system viewpoint, patients' values are a part of what they bring into the group. When therapist-leaders ask the people in activitiy groups to participate, values conflicts may result. For instance, people may be asked to play, even though they see play as something reserved for children, and not a valuable use of their time. Therapists may ask group members to engage in activities in which they touch or are touched, and this may seem an intimacy that should be reserved for family only. Therapists may ask group participants to put aside their intellect and "go with their feelings" when being intellectual is the only way some members have known how to be seen as valuable. Discussion of values conflicts may be facilitated by the use of values surveys or clarification exercises, (see figure 3.2).

It is not always possible to ask people about their values before they enter a group. Even if one asks, a good deal of what is learned about people's values emerges slowly in the process of getting to know them. However, group leaders need to be sensitive to patients and understand that a patient's reluctance to participate in group experiences may relate to matters of value. Therapists who work with patients from socio-cultural groups different than their own need to learn about these patients' cultural values and customs, and facilitate experiences that respect cultural differences. It is not the intent of activity groups to change anyone's values. Rather, the therapist-leader tries to create an environment in which patients are enabled to identify and think about their values. During activity groups, participants can gain an understanding of the relationship between their values, current life satisfaction, and/or problems. Often it is just as important for individuals to consider and reaffirm their values as it is to question them, as they look ahead to the paths they hope to follow in their lives.

Values Survey

Directions: Please write your name and then place an X in front of those items that you value. Place your initials by those characteristics that you have personally, objects that you own, relationships that you have and goals that you are currently pursuing.

Name: _____

Valued Personal Characteristics

(Initials)

——	Honest	——
——	Friendly	——
——	Helpful	——
——	Polite	——
——	Obedient	——
——	Broad minded	——
——	Beauty	——
——	Intelligence	——

Valued Objects

(Initials)

——	Car	——
——	House	——
——	Books	——
——	Sports equipment	——
——	Boat	——
——	Clothes	——
——	Art Objects	——
——	Antiques	——
——	Musical instruments	——
——	Jewelry	——
——	Money	——

Valued Relationships:

(Initial)

——	Friends	——
——	Spouse	——
——	Parents	——
——	Children	——
——	Sexual relationship	——
——	Intimate relationship	——
——	Family (extended)	——
——	Neighbor	——

Other:

——
——
——

Valued Goals:

(Initial)

——	Education	——
——	Exciting life	——
——	Freedom from stress	——
——	Social recognition	——
——	Respect from peers	——
——	Financial security	——
——	Satisfying career	——
——	Health and physical comfort	——
——	World peace	——

Three most important values:

_____

_____

_____

Figure 3.2   Values Survey

The Social Situations Which Cause Patient Comfort or Discomfort

There are two major themes that repeat throughout therapy. One is that therapy has to involve some discomfort: change is not easy. The other is that when people are too uncomfortable or anxious, they resist change.

Beyond the fact that many people may be uncomfortable with the whole idea of change and the unknown expectations that lie ahead of them in therapeutic experiences, the small activity group adds an additional stress to the prospect of therapy. In small groups, members are asked to face the possibility of making public those personal problems with which they grapple. The idea of participating in activities that may be unfamiliar, with people they don't know, when they aren't feeling very good about themselves is not usually appealing to anyone.

Although group leaders can't eliminate all anxiety (nor should they try) there are some things they can do to help keep discomfort manageable.

It is often helpful to ask prospective group members about the kinds of group and social experiences they've had. Many persons get clammy palms just thinking about having to say anything within a group setting, or facing the prospect of being on a "team" (recalling their shame at not ever being selected for team play with peers when they were young). Student therapists and patients have reported their discomfort with having to "hold hands and form a circle" in various group exercises, yet how often have group leaders begun with this instruction? Some individuals feel uncomfortable with anything that seems groupy. They may describe themselves as "loners" or "best in a one-to-one relationship." Figure 3.3 is a brief survey of group experiences that might be discussed with prospective group participants. When there is not an opportunity to meet individually with group members, this survey can form the basis of a small group exercise or dialogue that can be carried out with the entire group.

Patient Social and Vocational Roles

Each patient brings multiple roles into the treatment setting. An individual may be a parent, son or daughter, housekeeper, computer operater, church member, and so on, depending on the social or vocational setting in which each finds him or herself. These roles serve as input or backgound to the group. We often ask patients about their vocational and avocational roles when we talk with them about their social experiences.

Survey of Group Experiences

Name: _____   Date: _____

Please place a check in the space provided by those groups in which you have participated. Give brief answers to all other questions.

Groups in which you have been a member:
_____ Family
_____ Church
_____ Community
_____ Work
_____ Professional organization
_____ Neighborhood
_____ Peer
_____ School
_____ Social clubs
_____ Other: _____

Treatment groups in which you have participated:
_____ Occupational therapy
_____ Recreational therapy
_____ Social skills training
_____ Assertive training
_____ Family therapy
_____ Outpatient groups
_____ Art therapy
_____ Music therapy
_____ Dance therapy
_____ Other _____

When in a group, what role(s) do you like to assume?
(e.g active participant, observer, follower, leader)

_____

What do you like least about being in a group?

_____

What do you like best about being in a group?

_____

Please describe how a group has helped you.

_____

_____

_____

Figure 3.3   Survey of Group Experiences

Often this information influences the individual goals that they have in treatment. It is vital to recognize, however, that group and other treatment experiences can be a leveler, because the roles that patients have had at home and work are often unrecognized as they now assume the role of patient and group member. Small group activity meetings do not start with introductions such as "This is John, a plumber," or "This is Fran, a homemaker." It is not that familiar roles are lost but they are in a sense put on the back burner. This can be very disconcerting to persons who rely on those kind of role definitions in their relationships to other people.

Interaction Roles

In addition to social and vocational roles, individuals bring the group a preferred style of relating. For example, some people choose to be "laid back" when relating to others, others prefer to take charge. These inter-action styles can also be indentified as the patterns of behavior or roles that one takes. Interaction roles usually become more evident as the group progresses and become a part of the group's throughput or process. Interaction roles are discussed in more detail in chapter 8.

Initally therapist-leaders may want to enhance the patients' opportu-nity to assume particular group roles. For instance, the person who likes to be the leader's helper might be asked to be in charge of getting equipment or seating arranged; the person who likes to sit back and observe might well be allowed to do so until their comfort level supports increased group participation.

One other element that influences how comfortable patients are in various kinds of social situations is the activity that is in progress in a particular group. Activites are discussed further in the next chapter.

The Enabling Group Climate

While therapists hope that the small activity group can provide a positive or relearning experience, it cannot do so unless patients know that they will not be forced to engage in an activity or behave in a manner that will be terribly anxiety-producing for them. Group leaders can validate the patients' feelings, and try to begin with group activities that respect the level of social skills most consistent with the group members' ability. If, for example, most of the group members have trouble with closeness, try not to force disclosure and touching. Rather, start by selecting an activity that asks for only superficial contact, cooperation, and/or sharing.

It is not true, in our experience, that something that is beneficial always has to hurt or taste bad, but moving out of the status quo does necessitate some risk. Therapists need to create a supportive setting in which participants who are ready to manage some anxiety or discomfort can try out new roles within the group, new ways of experiencing and expressing feelings, new skills, or unfamiliar ideas. One way to enable risk taking is for leaders to assure patients that they understand that the group experience can be uncomfortable, and that if group members need to be involved only minimally or sporadically, their need will be respected. Therapists let members know that the choice to try something uncomfortable must be theirs, and that they don't need to take risks to please therapists or to get approval. For example: "Frank, I see that you've been pretty reluctant to get involved today. I can tell that this activity was hard for you. I want you to know that I won't push you to do something that doesn't feel right to you. I still value you as a group member. Maybe another time you might want to try this activity. Please stay in the group, and participate and contribute to the extent you are able."

The Patient's Ability to be Active, Organized and Effectively Boundaried

We said earlier that these three components spoke directly to the patient's ability to participate in the group activity, and the therapist will want to be cognizant of the prospective group member's skills in this area.

Active Participation

The ability to be *active* refers to the level of energy that the patient has and is willing and able to invest in the group.

The concept of open systems presumes that people have the energy available to meet their needs. The fact is, however, that persons who are physically ill, persons who are elderly and have been sitting around in non-stimulating settings, persons who are distressed by emotional problems, and others may not come into the group with much available energy. When group members lack energy, it is often the group leader who needs to bring surplus energy and infuse it into the activity to increase and support patient participation. The following are some familiar concepts that can be used to assess an individual's ability to be an active group participant.

Motivation — Does the patient demonstrate a desire to be in the group? Arrive at group independently? On time?

Arousal — Does the patient express enthusiasm for the activity? The group? Does the patient demonstrate pleasure/enthusiasm when relating to group members?

Energy level — Does the patient's physical body suggest he/she is alert? lethargic? agitated? drained? hyperactive (with excesssive or random activity)?

Awareness — Does the patient seem aware of what is going on in the group setting? Does he/she demonstrate an understanding of what behaviors are expected, and what is available to the patient in the group?

Assertiveness/Passivity — Can the person ask for what he or she needs, or appropriately take what is needed from within the group? Can patients stand up for what they believe or value? Do they allow unpleasant things to happen to them? Do they wait to be noticed?

Frustration Tolerance — Does the patient complain of being nervous? Make frequent requests to leave the group and return to his or her room? Are patients unable to sit during the group? Do they pace? Smoke excessively (if allowed to smoke during treatment)? Are they easily irritated by group members? the leader? the activity experience?

Patient Organization

In system language, *organization* addresses the individual's ability to make sense of personal experience, and to plan action so that tasks can be carried out from start to completion. In terms of organization one considers:

Discrimination — Can the person recognize the salient features of a problem, situation, or task?

Concept Formation — Does the patient appear able to create a mental picture of what is expected of him or her and what action is being called for?

Organization of materials — Can the person obtain and organize tools and other media as needed in tasks?

Memory — Does the person have an adequate memory to sustain activity involvement?

Goal Directed Behavior — Does the person seem to know where to begin when starting an activity? Can he or she make choices or decisions as needed? Can he or she carry an activity from start to finish? If not, what seems to get in the way of goal completion?

Patient Boundaries

Boundaries refer to conceptual limits that keep seperate what exists within and outside the self. Flexible boundaries allow the patient to effectively give and take within a changing environment while maintaining a sense of the self's integrity. Boundaries are also demonstrated in the individual's ability for reality testing and to exert self-control. Some familiar terms used in relation to boundaries are:

Reality orientation — Do patients have a realistic idea of why they are in treatment? Are they aware of time, place, and circumstance?

Thought disorder — Is there indication of severely distorted thinking; for example, hallucinations, ideas of reference, or confusion?

Detail — When involved in an activity, can the patient give adequate attention to details so that activity can be accomplished? Or, does over attention to detail get the patient "stuck" somewhere in the process?

Self-image — Does the person see him or herself as real and meaningful? Can he or she separate his or her ideas from those of others? Is self-assessment reasonably accurate (a subjective judgment)? Is the person able to set realistic goals?

Openness — Is the person able to consider new ideas or ways of doing things? Will he or she let others get to know them?

Flooding — Does the patient appear overwhelmed by contact, feedback or other information coming into the self?

Flexibility — Can the patient tolerate and adapt to a change in plans? Can he or she compromise without a fear of loss of self identity or esteem?

Assessing the Patient Group System

Thus far, we have considered the individual patient's values, strengths and limitations, history of group experiences, energy level and functional abilities that serve as guiding concepts for working in a group setting. These concepts and individual patient considerations are further developed by group leaders to evaluate how the patients can be expected to work together in the group. Getting this larger picture enables leaders to make knowledgeable decisions about which group format to choose, what kind of activities to use, and how best to participate as leader.

The following is our modification of a milieu assessment used by Hoffman-Grotting at UCLA Neuropsychiatric Institute, Los Angeles. The therapist working in a setting where there is a rapid turnover of patients can come each morning and look through the cardex, or other summary of the patient population, then use this form as a guide to conceptualize the group membership as a whole. Therapists working in a setting where the patient population remains more stable might use such a guide only infrequently.

Milieu Assessment

Unit: ——————   **Date:** ————

Therapist: ——————————————

Census:

    Setting
    Focus of services
    Average length of stay

Patient/Resident Descriptors:

    Age clusters
    Diagnostic categories (physical or psycho-social)
    Social roles
    Performance problems

Milieu Characteristics:

    Significant events impacting the unit

Precautions:

Weekly Recommendations:

Figure 3.4a   Milieu Assessment Guide

Milieu Assessment		

Unit: ___Geropsychiatry___ Date: ___8-21-88___ Therapist: ___S.S.___

Census:

    Total ___22___   Male ___5___   Female ___17___

Patient/Resident Descriptors:

Age Clusters:

    Age 56-65 ___5___
    Age 66-75 ___12___
    Age 75-85 ___5___

Diagnostic Categories: (May be psycho-social or physical disorders)

Developmental Disorder	1	Rheumatoid Arthritis	4
Organic Mental Disorder	10	Diabetic	12
Psychotic Disorder	6	Cardiac	4
Mood Disorder	15	CVA	2
Alzeheimer's	1	Renal Disease	2

Social Roles:
    Worker _____   Retiree __X__   Other: __Nursing Home__
                        Homaker __X__   __Resident__

Performance Problems:

Vision	1 legally blind	Self care	8 need assistance
Auditory	X	Vocational	
Motor	———	Recreational/leisure	X
Sensory	———	Social Roles	
Tactile	———	Communication	X (75% withdrawn)
Cognitive	X	Problem solving	X (dependent in)

Milieu Characteristics:

    Many disoriented patients; very short attention spans
    Nursing staff shortage

Significant Events:

    Patient had cardiac arrest and expired two nights ago.
    Patients talking about death.
    Staff discussing the event and the protocol followed.
    Several doctors away on vacation.

Precautions:
        3 persons on suicide precautions

        diet restrictions

Weekly Recommendations:

Figure 3.4b   Milieu Assessment Sample

Chapter Summary

The emphasis in this chapter has been on two dimensions of input into the group's system: that of the treatment environment and of those individuals who will make up the treatment group.

The environment, or milieu, is recognized for the physical boundaries and background information it provides, as well as the emotional messages it gives. In large part, the milieu is created by the patient group. Each patient brings into the group experience a personal history of strengths, limitations, preferences and expectations. While we don't propose one specific patient screening tool, we have found in our own experience that it is useful to gain an understanding of each prospective participant's (a) beliefs regarding why they are in treatment, (b) strengths, (c) values, (d) comfort with social situations, and (e) specific skills related to the ability to be active, organized and boundaried within a group.

On a day to day basis, the milieu is viewed as ever changing or as being re-created as new experiences impact the treatment setting and the patient group as a whole.

4
Group Input: The Activity

Focus Questions

1. How can activity arouse and sustain interest?
2. What are the twelve dimensions of activity?
3. What provides boundaries within a group activity experience?
4. What is the activity group?
5. What characteristics of the therapist-leader will influence the group experience and outcome?
6. What is the relationship between the therapist's frame of reference and the use of activity?
7. What is the difference between a generalized versus a personalized approach to activity analysis?

Activity as a System of Participation

The thing that most clearly distinguishes therapeutic activity groups from other small therapy groups is the planned use of activity. When people are active, they are "doing something." And, as used in this text, they are doing something beyond just talking. In the latter portion of this book, there are many examples of therapeutic activity groups. The activities described are purposeful, planned, and lend themselves to group participation and the achievement of therapeutic goals.

People's choice of words, their language, tells much about what they value . If a person says, "I was active in the Girl Scouts when I was young," or "I'm active in my community," it is implied that their participation in these groups was important. Passivity is the opposite of activity, and it tends to imply inertia. Being active carries with it the notion of one's reaching out and having impact. That is, rather than something being done to the person, he or she is the participant. Rather than having choices made for them, they are required to make choices. If being passive suggests the saving of energy, being active connotes its expenditure.

The Dimensions of Activity

When therapists ask patients to expend energy in therapeutic groups, they need to have clear ideas about what makes activity both appealing and useful. In this book, therapeutic activity is cited as having twelve key dimensions.

1. It is capable of arousing and sustaining interest.
2. It allows participants to take responsibility.
3. It has a purpose (or aim).
4. It requires an investment of energy from participants.
5. It has relevance to the persons involved in it.
6. It is viewed as therapeutic by the therapist using it, and it is tied to an acceptable therapeutic theory and practice base.
7. It is a system with an organization that includes rules or techniques (methodologies), and sometimes equipment, objects and tools.
8. It is a system that takes on meaning from its interrelationship with individual, socio-cultural, and treatment systems.
9. It has a start and a finish.
10. It is a system that can be analyzed in terms of demands on the physical, spiritual, psychological, social, and cognitive parts of of the person-system.
11. It has boundaries as established by the person system and the nature of the activity process.
12. It strives to strike a balance between demands and the patient's capability and committment to involvment.

You, the reader may want to add to this list, depending upon your own view of therapeutic activity. Cynkin suggests, for example, that for activity to be therapeutic, it also needs to be practical and versatile in order to meet the real, day-to-day demands in the treatment setting (Cynkin 1979, 48). The twelve dimensions listed are inexorably related, and deserve further discussion.

Therapeutic Activity Can Arouse and Sustain Interest

Sensory Arousal

When people describe something as being "arousing" we tend in our culture to think of its sensual qualities. That is, it catches our attention, perhaps in its brightness, harsh touch or strong smell. While sensory arousal is one way that activities can alert the person, it is only one of several levels of arousal used by therapists in their daily work. Activities that appeal to the five senses can be conceived developmentally as depending upon a lower level of arousal, since they do not appeal initially to conscious thought processes. This level of arousal may be used appropriately when group participants are functioning at a low cognitive level. For instance: Ross and Burdick (1981,39) describe the initial stage of an activity group designed for chronic, regressed adults. First, the patients are placed in a circle, and a vibrator is offered to each one. Then, a heavy metal bell is introduced by the therapist who rings the bell says her own name, and then asks each participant to do the same, and passes the bell along. Finally, a puffy, red powder puff is used on the members' arms or lightly on their cheeks and then passed along. These sensory experiences are designed to get attention, to alert the patient system, and to begin to evoke some associations, and/or small, positive interest.

The limitation of sensory arousal is that it can not sustain interest over long periods. Put most simply, people either become irritated or worn out by it if they are overexposed.

Play and Exploration

The next level of arousal, one capable of sustaining interest for longer periods, is arousal related to simple play and exploration. This kind of arousal appeals to human curiosity, and the joy that persons can experience from using their bodies, feelings, and/or thoughts to try new things. For example, a group in the community recently offered a yoga class directed towards the "over fifty" crowd. Several of the participants said that they were drawn to the activity because it was something they had heard about and "always wanted to try."

Learning and Mastery

Once an individual tries something new, it isn't new anymore. Hence, to keep their interest, the activity must eventually move beyond the novel. It sustains the individual's interest because it provides an opportunity for learning and eventual mastery. For example, if a person becomes involved in a weaving group, he or she does not necessarily leave the group upon having learned the first weaving pattern; rather, involvement is sustained when new weavers perceive themselves as adding to their skills, when they see their accomplishments, and can picture themselves as becoming adept at weaving. Activity that sustains interest in this way is activity that provides an opportunity for education. It allows participants to not only find out what they can accomplish, but also to learn what they can't do. In this way activity enables individuals to learn about their boundaries in relation to their world.

Value and Relevance of Activity

Activity is capable of holding people's interest when it appeals to their values.

An activity group at the local elder center involved the members getting together to watch the presidential debates, and having a post-debate dialogue. This activity group had some obvious sensory-arousal capacity; the hoots and hollers of the group was far more boisterous than the controlled tenor of the candidates themselves.

There was an element of novelty, in that presidential elections come along only every four years. Some individuals stopped and watched only briefly responding to their curiosity about what was going on, but not choosing to stay with the group. Those who sustained their involvement did so because they had the opportunity to voice ideas that were important to them in terms of their values. In voicing their support for their candidate, group participants gave expression to significant personal beliefs.

Another reason that this group activity was able to hold group interest was that group members perceived it as relevant. The choice of a new president was taken very seriously by many members of the group. They listened for clues in the debate about both candidates' plans for health care, Social Security, and taxes.

In summary, activity will catch and maintain a person's interest only when it matches the individual's own developmental needs. For the most part, group members need to be able to see in the group activity something they can and want to get for themselves. This need for self gratification and fulfillment can be explored further when considering the activity's purpose.

Therapeutic Activity Gives Participants Responsibility

Therapeutic activity is not a spectator sport. While many prospective participants may choose to begin their participation cautiously, even as observers, or may need the therapist to initially structure their participation, the goal in therapeutic activity is to enable patients to make decisions, to participate, and to take responsibility for what they do in the activity. People can experience some vicarious pleasure in seeing the fun others are having or can vicariously identify with others' frustration. Studies in modeling and role acquisition indicate that people can learn from their observation of others (Bandura 1971, 1977). But, if they as individuals are to enhance their own self-worth and gain a sense of personal mastery regarding specific skills, they need to engage as active participants. In addition, it is only as active participants that patients can receive the feedback and validation that the group context for therapeutic activity can offer.

Therapeutic Activity has an Identifiable Purpose

In order for activity to be therapeutic, it must successfully bond the goals of therapy with the nature of the activity itself.

Some of the activities used for therapy are those commonly associated with work. In this case, work is defined broadly as the expenditure of energy to provide food, shelter, or clothing; and not in its stricter definition as activity that generates income (Burrus-Bammell, 1982, 123).

Other activities commonly used in therapy are those associated with physical exercise, self-care and maintenance, and leisure and recreation. Many therapeutic activities do not fit into such neat little boxes. For example, those activities designed to increase self-awareness, to clarify values, or to enhance creative expression have multiple purposes and varied approaches to meet identified goals.

Regardless of the type of activity, the therapist and patient need to be clear about its purpose. The activity may have a purpose because it involves a specific task to be accomplished or skill to be gained, or because it otherwise relates directly to one of the therapeutic goals that have been selected and identified for the patient.

Some of the most frequently cited goals of therapeutic activities are identified in the following (not to be construed as an exhaustive list):

- to provide needed boundaries
- to enhance self-esteem, self identity, confidence and control
- to enhance the development of specific task skills
- to provide an alternative to stressful situations
- to increase opportunity for social skill building
- to facilitate recreation and play
- to allow for creativity and self-expression
- to provide a means for education (including knowledge building and information sharing)
- to provide an opportunity for intermember support and to increase a feeling of community
- to build cognitive awareness and/or to reinforce reality
- to give members a chance to contribute to the larger community.

Purpose Related to the Therapist's Frame of Reference

When activity is used in the therapeutic context it must fit with the specific principles of therapy as applied by the therapist. These *frames of reference* are the guiding beliefs about health and health care that enable therapists to make responsible practice decisions. Frames of reference exist that emphasize the person-system as an individual; (e.g., theoretical models related to neuroanatomy and physiology; personality theories such as those of behaviorism, developmental theory, cognitive and object-relations theories).

Other theoretical frameworks emphasize the group and group process; (e.g., gestalt, T-groups, encounter groups, milieu therapy). These would concern themselves with the creation of group norms for behavior, leadership styles, role division within groups, etc. There are also theories that emphasize the person in the family; (e.g. family-system theories and intervention models).

The frame of reference that is selected by the therapist-leader may be *eclectic* and may represent a synthesis of theory related to the individual, group, and society at large, but it should nevertheless be based upon accepted methodologies and a firm knowledge base. This guiding frame of reference not only grounds the therapist in his or her practice, it allows for the cogent sharing of information with other professionals, and for the effective adaptation of activity.

There are countless ways to use a specific activity or medium effectively, and more than one activity that could be selected to meet a specified group need at any given time. Being able to structure and present a given activity in a way that is most beneficial to the needs of an identified treatment group is the essence of activity as therapy.

The following serves as an example of how the same activity, (drawing the self) might be used in three different ways, towards three different ends, depending on the needs of the participants and the theory base guiding practice.

Activity: Drawing the Self

Experience A: In a cognitive rehabilitation group, composed mostly of recovering stroke patients, the therapist asks a group member to lean against the wall where a large piece of paper has been attached. Someone traces around their body form. Patients are then asked to draw in where the various body parts, clothes, etc., would go.

Experience B: In a self awareness group, composed of adolescent girls, each participant is asked to use a pencil to draw a portrait of themselves on a piece of 8x11 inch paper. The therapist leads a discussion that focuses on body-image concerns.

Experience C: In a communication group composed of identified patients and their families, the group participants are asked to draw a picture of themselves along with other family members. The therapeutic discussion/processing stresses family dynamics.

The Immediacy of Therapeutic Activity

If one considers the therapeutic aim of the activity as the broad or 'macra' purpose, there must still exist a more immediate sense of purpose. In other words, patients coming into the activity need to know that what they are being asked to do has an identifiable goal that can be achieved within the activity period. This is facilitated when the therapist makes clear that the activity has a start, a process, and a conclusion within the group's meeting. Much of this is accomplished by the therapist's introductory comments to the group and the use of specific process observations during and at the conclusion of the group session. For example, the therapist may say, "Welcome. It's nice to see all of you again. If you remember, the last time we met we decided that today's session would be used to write a mock resume so that those of you getting ready to get a job can practice summarizing your employment history and selling your knowledge and skills on paper. I know that for some of you this is "old hat" and it would be really helpful if you could share your expertise with the group. Since we have our usual 45 minutes, let's plan to stop at quarter 'til eleven. That'll give us time to review what we've accomplished, and still have a few minutes to share the snack that Joan brought us." (Then, when closing,) "Well, it's 10:45 and it's time to begin our wrap-up. Tom, thank you for volunteering your work history for the group to practice resume writing. I think by stressing the skills that you used in each of your jobs, we've worked up a resume that would let any employer know what a good resource he'd have if he hired you! I was really impressed by the creativity that the group showed today. You've come up with many useful and, I think, sensitive ideas to help you as you respond to employer biases about hiring people with physical limitations. (Pause for a response.) Now, please share your reactions to today's group. Or tell what you achieved or gained during the last hour."

In summary, the purpose of the activity exists at two main levels: the larger aim as identified by the patient's goals and consistent with the theoretical frame of reference, and the more immediate, goal-directednature of an activity that has a start, a process, and an identifiable conclusion. These characteristics help establish the relevance of the activity for each group member. In the above employment (resume) group, the larger aim is employment preparation. The immediate activity goal is to produce an end product, (a resume) and gain skill practice in writing a resume.

Therapeutic Activity has Relevance to the Participant

It is one thing for an activity to be purposeful and goal-directed, but it may not be sufficient if the patient or patient group fails to see the relevance of the activity to their specific needs. If, for example, there are a group of older people sitting in the dayroom of a care facility, and the therapist suggests they join in a group to bake cookies, it would not be unusual to get a response like,"Why should I come? I can't eat anything with sugar anyway," or"Nothing tastes right to me anymore." Implied is the challenge, "What's in it for me?"

Another typical exchange occurs when the therapist asks a group of adolescents to express their feelings in a group collage. Some respond with, "Why should I? My problem is with my parents (or my school, or whomever), not with my friends, and your collage idea sounds stupid."

In our view, one of the primary reasons that patients may resist an activity group is that the group relevance to patient goals may not have been established. As with the examples previously used, the patient group needs to know why baking cookies is a beneficial activity for them (if indeed it is). For example, it might be stressed that when they share an experience, they learn to work together and make a contribution to holiday festivities. Or when adolescents work on a group collage, there can be a link between sharing feelings common to all adolescents and learning alternative ways to relate to parents and other authority figures.

Broadly speaking, activities are more likely to be perceived as relevant when (a) they are consistent with what individuals value, (b) they are seen as a way to learn something that the person wants to know, (c) they are valued by the person's peers or those with whom he or she identifies, and (d) they fit with what the individual feels is a need in the here-and-now.

The Therapist's View of Therapeutic Activity

Different therapists may select different kinds of activities to be used in the group, in part because of differing patient goals and abilities, and in part because of the therapist's own preferences. Whatever activity is used, patients and staff can sense the therapist's belief in the value of the activity. When therapists believe in an activity, they communicate that the activity is worthwhile and can lead to goal attainment. This can be especially significant when a patient is unfamiliar with the planned activity, or his or her energy and motivation are in short supply.

Therapeutic Activity: A System with Component Parts

Playing a game of checkers, reading the newspaper, participating in a group sing-along, riding an exercycle, building a playhouse — all activities — make different demands of the person system, and have different component parts as a system in itself. Because of the diverse range of activities used in therapy groups and the multiple purposes for using a particular activity, it is difficult to find one best way to catalog the activities and their purpose or to analyze their component parts and relationships. However, from a system perspective, there are three key elements of an activity to consider: the demands of the activity, the personal meaning of the activity and the activity's boundaries.

Activity Demands

One of the traditional approaches is to look at the demands that the activity makes on each part of the person system. For instance, the physical demands of the activity can be judged by looking at what is required of body mechanics, range of motion of specific joints, muscle strength, overall physical endurance, sensory-motor coordination, etc. Cognitive demands can be evaluated in relation to the developmental level of problem solving used, the requirements relative to attention, concentration, and short-term, procedural or other modes of memory storage, and recall. Activities also have social-emotional demands which are expressed in the requirements for creativity, self expression, and personal interaction. Figure 4.1 entitled Analyzing Activity depicts this approach to activity analysis.

Analyzing activity in this way has its limitations. One of the biggest drawbacks is that it fails to leave room for the idea that activity need not have any absolute qualities (or that activity is different each time another person applies their own unique stamp to it, or gives it personal meaning based on their life experiences.)

Personal Meaning of Activity

Cynkin refers to the personalizing of activity as its "acquired properties," (Cynkin 1979, 123). Thus, in a manner more consistent with general system theory, the actions, objects, relationships, and symbolic referents of the activity are assessed in relation to each participant; his or her special

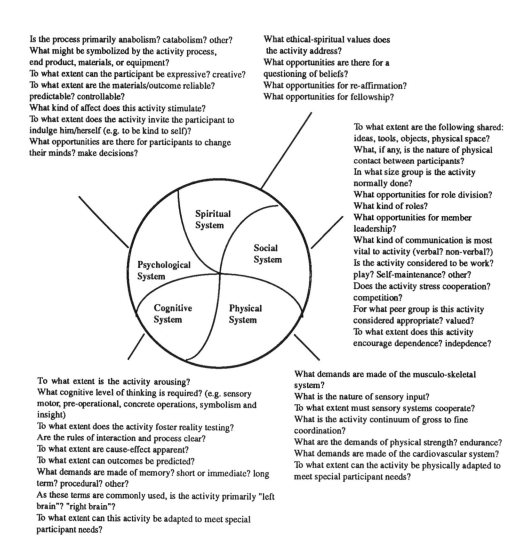

Is the process primarily anabolism? catabolism? other?
What might be symbolized by the activity process,
end product, materials, or equipment?
To what extent can the participant be expressive? creative?
To what extent are the materials/outcome reliable?
predictable? controllable?
What kind of affect does this activity stimulate?
To what extent does the activity invite the participant to
indulge him/herself (e.g. to be kind to self)?
What opportunities are there for participants to change
their minds? make decisions?

What ethical-spiritual values does
the activity address?
What opportunities are there for a
questioning of beliefs?
What opportunities for re-affirmation?
What opportunities for fellowship?

To what extent are the following shared:
ideas, tools, objects, physical space?
What, if any, is the nature of physical
contact between participants?
In what size group is the activity
normally done?
What opportunities for role division?
What kind of roles?
What opportunities for member
leadership?
What kind of communication is most
vital to activity (verbal? non-verbal?)
Is the activity considered to be work?
play? Self-maintenance? other?
Does the activity stress cooperation?
competition?
For what peer group is this activity
considered appropriate? valued?
To what extent does this activity
encourage dependence? indepdence?

To what extent is the activity arousing?
What cognitive level of thinking is required? (e.g. sensory
motor, pre-operational, concrete operations, symbolism and
insight)
To what extent does the activity foster reality testing?
Are the rules of interaction and process clear?
To what extent are cause-effect apparent?
To what extent can outcomes be predicted?
What demands are made of memory? short or immediate? long
term? procedural? other?
As these terms are commonly used, is the activity primarily "left
brain"? "right brain"?
To what extent can this activity be adapted to meet special
participant needs?

What demands are made of the musculo-skeletal
system?
What is the nature of sensory input?
To what extent must sensory systems cooperate?
What is the activity continuum of gross to fine
coordination?
What are the demands of physical strength? endurance?
What demands are made of the cardiovascular system?
To what extent can the activity be physically adapted to
meet special participant needs?

Figure 4.1 Analyzing Activity

way of accomplishing the task process, his or her feelings about the activity,
the relationship of the activity to the individual's own roles and habits, and
all else that pertains to the personal relevance of the activity to the individual. Figure 4.2 proposes a format for what is referred to as a "personalized activity analysis." Such an analysis can be done by the therapist
spending time with each participant to assess the individual's personal
relationship with the activity process. This discussion may be between
patient and therapist or may occur during a treatment group when the
group leader and participants process an activity and summarize the
meaning of the group experience. (Activity processing is discussed in more
detail in chapter 6.)

Following the system model, in group activity, the therapist recognizes

---

Personalized Activity Analysis

Participant's Name:

Activity:

Does participant state he/she is familiar with this activity?
From where?

Does participant have experience with this activity? Briefly
describe.

Portions or attributes of activity participant states he/she
prefers:

Portion or attributes of activity participant states he is less
familiar or less comfortable with:

Does the participant view this activity as vocation/daily
maintenance/leisure/spiritual development/physical
exercise/social vehicle/combination?

Participants stated feelings/attitudes towards this activity:

Are therapist's observations of patient in activity (if
observation has occurred) congruent with what patient says
about his/her own involvement or attitude? Comment.

Figure 4.2   Personalized Activity Analysis

that the activity takes on meaning through its relationships with the patient,
with the group as a whole, and with the therapeutic milieu. The meaning
of activity is also influenced by the potential relationship it has with the
patient's community and the environment.

Activity: A System with Boundaries

When activity is carried out in a therapy group, there are a number
of parameters that separate or distinguish the activity from whatever else
may be going on in the treatment setting. The activity starts when the group
starts or when the leader and membership determine; it typically is carried
out within an identified time period; it is accomplished in an identified
physical space, and often necessitates specific supplies, tools or objects.
Either in a formal or informal way, it carries with it a set of procedures

or expectations for accomplishing the activity, and suggests auxillary behaviors which are acceptable during the process. All of this contributes to the activity's boundaries.

When the boundaries are specific, unambiguous and inflexible, the participants have specific information about the activity process and the behavioral expectations during the activity. As a result, the group participants have to make few choices and decisions. When patients are confused or particularly anxious, these clear boundaries can help orient them to their surroundings, guide their behavior to meet environmental expectations, and limit or reduce the stress of decision-making.

The more specific and defined the boundaries, the less opportunity there is for patient members to be creative or spontaneous in their participation. Obviously, depending on the nature of the patient group, the therapist may aim for more or less ambiguity and flexibility within the group and will select an activity that best meets patient needs and the therapeutic goals of the activity experience.

Reader Activity

The following three activity group experiences represent a continuum of activity boundaries, that demonstrate the relationship of boundaries to group goals and member characteristics.

Group A: The first group is one described in the *New Games Book.* New games are conceived as an alternative to the more rigid, highly competitive games played in the United States. In new games, participants often play out-of-doors or in another open environment. These games encourage the use of imagination, have flexible rules, ask for everyone's participation and strive for fun and a sense of celebration.

Group Experience: The Caterpillar

This group is described as a "delightful way to knock elbows, knees, heads and hips with your neighbor." The instructions are, get everyone lying on their stomachs, side-by-side. Make sure you're packed really closely together, and have little people squeeze between two big ones. Now have the person on the end of the line roll over onto her neighbor and keep rolling down the corduroy row of bodies. When she gets to the end of the line, she lies on her stomach, and the next person at the end of the line starts rolling. Once you get the momentum going, there'll be no stopping you, as your human caterpillar advances over meadows and hills (Flugelman 1976, 117).

Now, think about the boundaries described in the Group A experience. Ask yourself:

- Is there a time limit?
- Is there a limit to the number of participants?
- Is there a clear message regarding the behavior expected?
- What are the confines of the space in which the activity occurs?
- When is the activity finished?
- What are the boundaries of physical space between participants?
- What are the cognitive boundaries?
- What kind of patient group do you think could profit from the activity?
- For whom might it be contraindicated?

Group B: The second example is one frequently described in the literature (Ingersall and Goodman 1983; Butler 1980–81; Corey and Corey 1987) and one probably familiar to the therapists working with older adults. It is often referred to as a "reminiscence group." The themes in such a group are often isolation and loneliness, and the struggle to find meaning in life. The goals of these groups are to stimulate remembering, concentration, the building of affective associations, and social interaction. In the group described, the goal was not only to simulate reminiscence, but also to encourage recognition and discussion of change or how things are different today.

Group Experience: War of the Worlds

This group experience was one of an ongoing number of activity sessions designed to address the needs of an older population whose primary physical limitations were mild to moderate. The group met for 45 minutes, but this portion of the group was intended to last only 25 minutes. The remainder of the group was spent as it was in every session with a brief warm-up exercise and a snack at closing. Group membership was maintained at ten or less as small group atmosphere was as important to the achievement of group goals.

Members were seated in comfortable chairs, roughly in a semi-circle, and as close as possible to a tape recorder. The participants were instructed to listen closely and see if they could identify what they were about to hear. Then, they were asked to recall where they were, and what they remembered of their own experiences when the orginal was played as a radio broadcast nearly fifty years ago. About 10 minutes of Orson Wells' recital of the "War of the Words" was played. A group dialogue facilitated by the therapist-leader followed.

Now, think about how the boundaries of this group compared to those of Group A. Ask yourself:

- Is there a time limit?
- Is there a limit to the number of participants?
- Is there a clear message about the behavior expected?
- What are the confines of space in which activity occurs?
- When is the activity finished?
- Is there a limit to the number of participants?
- Are there cognitive boundaries? (Does this activity encourage imaginative thinking? Does it focus attention?)
- Which patient groups would benefit from this activity? For whom might it be contraindicated?

Group C: The third group is one designed to teach daily living skills to adults with developmental disabilities. It is described by Nochajski and Gordon (1987). Eight developmentally disabled adults were selected. The goal of the group was to teach functional living skills to the participants in a way that would be novel and rewarding, age-appropriate, and appealing.

Group Experience: Trivial Pursuit

In this group, members met for one hour per week, for eight sessions, to play an adapted version of the board game, Trivial Pursuit. A series of questions was developed by the therapist-leader in the following categories: functional signs, domestics/measurements, health and safety, time and money, social skills, and public services and occupations. Materials required included the Trivial Pursuit game board and pieces, a clock with movable hands, coins and bills, a telephone, and other functional skill items. The play ensued much as it does in the original game, with some modifications:

- The therapist reads the questions;
- Each player takes only one turn at a time, regardless of whether or not his or her answer is correct;
- If a player lands on a category in which he or she has already had a question, it will be his or her option to choose another category;

- The therapist encourages a group discussion after each answer;
- The therapist may prompt or cue the players having difficulty;
- If the therapy session ends before a player has all six colored pieces, the player with the most pieces wins.

Again, compare the boundaries of this activity to those preceding. Ask yourself:

- Is there a time limit?
- Is there a clear message regarding the behavior expected?
- What are the physical boundaries?
- How do the rules of the game contribute to the boundaries?
- Is there a limit on the number of participants?
- What are the cognitive boundaries?
- What kind of patient group could profit from this activity?
- For whom might it be ill-advised?

Energy to Engage in Therapeutic Activity

Freud proposed that as persons we have a limited (not endless) amount of energy, which he called libido. He said that if we invested most of our energy in one place, we would have little left over to put into other tasks. This idea can be represented by the person who puts all of his energy into work and comes home too tired to spend time (and energy) with his family.

Jung, more like von Bertalanffy, saw human beings as open energy systems. Both men proposed that energy flows into, through, and out of, the system in its constant exchanges with the environment. This idea could be represented by the way people feel "energized" by a particularly happy or successful experience.

Because the energy referred to here is not a commodity like dollars or gallons of gasoline, it remains beyond science's ability at this time to state how much energy is actually used in human activity. However, it seems safe to suggest that human participation in therapeutic activity does require an expenditure of energy. And, helpers who work with people in therapy often find that their patients seem to either lack or have problems drawing upon the energy needed to participate fully in the therapeutic activity. In chapter 9 we describe strategies which can help a leader mobilize an activity group that seems to lack energy.

Activity Demands Match Patient Readiness

Implicit in all of what has been discussed is that for activity to be therapeutic it must be compatible with what patients are capable of and ready to try.

The patients seen in treatment may or may not recognize their own skills. Either overestimating or underestimating their own abilities and limitations can be problematic. Being able to perceive latent skills, being able to assess readiness, understanding the demands made by activity, and appreciating the significance of the environment are all therapist responsibilities. This is further enhanced when the therapist establishes a sound therapeutic alliance with his or her patients, and creates an atmosphere in which patients do not have to feel overly anxious about possible mistakes that they might make. There is also the element of emotional readiness. The therapist involved in activity has many wonderful opportunities to be less than perfect, to join in an atmosphere of exploration, and at times sheer play, and can thereby help to free up energy for his or her group. But, if patients do not feel in a playful mood, then activities that respect or highlight their more somber thoughts might be far more fitting. When therapists select activities that are compatible with the patients' emotional readiness, the message conveyed is, "I am trying to understand your needs, and I accept you for who you are."

Chapter Summary

Therapeutic activity has been discussed as a system that makes demands on the whole person-participant. In order for the individual to realize the therapeutic potential of the group activity and to desire activity involvment, the activity must fit with the developmental needs and interests of that individual. As a system, activity has at least twelve (and possibly many more) dimensions that contribute to its ability to be used effectively in therapy. Summarized and for your review, the activity dimensions are:

1. It is capable of arousing and sustaining interest.

2. It allows participants to take responsibility.

3. It has a purpose or aim.

4. It requires an investment of energy from participants.

5. It has relevance to participants.

6. It is viewed as therapeutic by the therapist and tied to an acceptable therapeutic base.

7. It is a system with an organization that includes rules, techniques, and sometimes equipment, objects and tools.

8. It takes on meaning from its interrelationship with individual, social-cultural, and treatment systems.

9. It has a start and a finish.

10. It can be analyzed in terms of demands on the physical, spiritual, psychological, social, and cognitive parts of the person system.

11. It has boundaries.

12. It poses a balance between demands and the patient's capacity for and commitment to involvement.

5
Group Input: The Therapist

Focus Questions

1. What personal characteristics of the therapist influence his or her role in the group?
2. What professional characteristics of the therapist influence the therapist's interaction in the group?
3. What expectations do therapists have of group participants? Of themselves?

Therapist Characteristics — You as a System

The therapist, just like the patient and all persons, can be thought of as a vital system of feelings, beliefs and potentialities. As a system, the therapist embodies an organized structure that thrives on energy and is defined and limited by boundaries.

Self-Image

We can pause here and reflect on what self-image means to the individual. Each therapist has specific abilities gained through life experiences. Each has knowledge, plus a myriad of personal beliefs. When something new happens in a person's life, it is not typically experienced as random information. Rather, the individual gives it personal meaning according to the unique, personal structure of the self. Some refer to this organizing structure as the "self-image" or the"self-concept." It is also compatible with what has been referred to as a cognitive map, in which the person organizes information and experience into patterns. (Tolman 1932). Who we are as persons includes all abilities, beliefs and boundaries of which we are consciously aware as well as those that we describe as unconscious, yet integrated into our being. That information and those abilities that we are consciously aware of (or those of which we are "self-aware") enable us as therapists to choose how we will respond.

In 1973, encounter group leader William Schutz wrote, "You are a unified organism. You are at the same time physical, psychological, and spiritual. These levels are manifestations of the same essence. You function best when these aspects are integrated and when you are self aware". (Schutz 1973, 16).

It is important for therapists to recognize what they can and can not do well, and equally, to know how their personal beliefs color what they judge to be true, and direct their actions. One can think of the self-image as having a "selective permeability" (Liff 1979) in that persons tend to allow in only those perceptions that are consistent with the belief system that they already possess. Everything associated with the self-concept and personal cognitive maps that organize information contribute to therapist boundaries.

Therapist Self-Awareness

Years back, consistent with what was then the dominant Freudian influence in medicine, the discussion of self-awareness within the therapeutic relationship revolved around understanding transference and countertransference within the therapist-patient relationship. To elaborate, therapists expected patients to respond to them as if they were significant others in the patients lives eliciting a therapist response that conformed to the patient's expectations. Self-awareness as it is used here refers to a broader awareness by the therapist regarding all that he or she is and how he or she fits within the greater social and world systems. There is no magic route to self-awareness, although sitting around all day is among the least likely routes. What can be hoped for instead is the therapist's openness to a recognition of the significance of personal biases and expectations, the therapist's flexibility in assessment of the meaning of new experiences and the therapist's ability to evaluate the influence of these as they impact the group outcome and leadership style.

As you think of yourself as an activity group leader or prospective leader consider: a) your view of others, b) your personal strengths and limitations, c) the authority of your knowledge and expectations, d) the group and its outcome, and e) the role you have within the milieu.

View of Others

Closely related to one's view of others is the question "What do I think facilitates change?"

Therapists might be tempted to answer this in terms of their frame of reference: the personality theories and the treatment tenets to which they ascribe. However, the person's view of others and of the world began forming at birth, not in college. Helpers, just like all people, learn from their early experiences whether people are basically "good" or whether they need to be closely watched and guided to be kept out of trouble. Helpers, too, form strong impressions about how they can influence others and about the conditions in their own lives that encouraged (or discouraged) them in making certain choices.

Reader Activity

In order to clarify for yourself how your own values and biases may influence a group in which you are involved, try to answer the following: (The final four of these are suggested by Saretsky (1977) in his book *Active Techniques and Group Psychotherapy*)

1. Can my patients be trusted to take responsibility for themselves?
2. How do I see patients as different from myself? from other staff?
3. Are there certain people or groups of people that I see as more (or less) okay than others?
4. How do I think people learn best?
5. What patients have I gossiped about to a colleague?
6. If a particular patient is absent or late, do I ever fail to notice? Am I ever glad?
7. How would I like my troublesome or difficult patients to change?
8. Draw a picture of your group and tell a story about it.

Personal Strengths and Limitations

No one can do everything well. If people are fortunate, however, they have had a variety of experiences that have helped them to gain a sense of what they do well, where they need support or assistance, and when they are in over their heads. Having this information allows the person to channel his or her energy in ways that are compatible with self-image, and thereby supports the personal boundarying system.

Therapists can ask themselves,"What do I bring into the helping relationship, (here the group specifically) that represents a use of my special talents or abilities? In what kind of situations do I feel most at home? In what situations do I feel awkward or out of place? Where do I shine?

Many therapists who use activities therapeutically do so in part because of their love of the activity medium itself — be it music, dance, the graphic

graphic arts, sports or other. Their ability to communicate their belief in the intrinsic worth of the medium they use and their enthusiasm and energy for the activity and their patient's participation both enhance their therapy. Other therapists may have a less keen affection for any particular activity, but may, nonetheless, be able to recognize and use the attributes of activity in an effective way.

The effectiveness of varying therapeutic approaches is exemplified in the following developmental differences of two therapists.

Kelly is a student nurse who co-leads the activity group. The patients are obviously attracted to her enthusiasm, though some grumble that she is "too darn cheery." Kelly either hasn't read the patients' histories very closely, or she simply chooses not to believe that these patients are chronically disabled and can not be expected to change. She approaches all of them with the attitude that together they will have a productive group experience. Interestingly, many of these patients are participating in this group more actively and appropriately than they have in previous hospitalizations.

Daisy is a seasoned therapist, having seen her 55th birthday years ago. Patients are attracted to her also. They respond to her no-nonsense, yet caring approach. When she conducts a group, she lets the members know that life can be tough and she says that from personal experience — but that sitting around 'on our duffs' isn't going to help anything.

Two different personalities, two different approaches to therapy, yet both therapists are able to be effective group leaders. When therapists think about their own strengths and limitations as well as their beliefs, it is helpful if they consider themselves as evolving beings. They are not as they were three or seven or ten years ago. It is not that they take on a whole new personality, but new information is gained, new experiences internalized, and some ideas let go. At times it becomes a comparison of what is emphasized or seen as most important, and what seems disposable. Through all of this, there are many threads of continuity that maintain the system's wholeness.

Take a moment and think about your values and priorities seven to ten years ago, compared to those of the present. Are you aware of changes? Do these changes seem subtle or drastic? How have you changed or remained the same? Would people who knew you ten years ago know you today?

The Authority of Knowledge

Self-knowledge is not all therapists need to be competent leaders. It is knowledge of health and disability, of activity, of groups, and of much else that prepares the therapist to be a competent helper. Brill refers to this as the knowledge that enables authority. As she states, "Workers who do not possess more and better knowledge about how to deal with the concerns of their clients or the general public have no right to intervene in people's lives. Teachers must know their subjects and how to teach; doctors must know medicine and have skills in using this knowledge and so forth." (Brill 1985, 107).

With knowledge becoming so vast, therapist limitations become more apparent. An important part of all therapists' knowledge is reflected in their knowing where they are not well informed. Therapists are not equally trained or prepared in using the various therapeutic activity media, in working with specific groups or patient problems, or in using specific group formats. It is the therapists', ethical responsibility to keep their knowledge base and skills sound and up-to-date, and to work only in areas in which they have expertise. This ethical responsibility serves as another boundary to the therapist-system.

Expectations of the Group Experience

It is essential that all helpers realize that they, too, gain something from their work as group leaders and therapists. For many it is that 'good feeling' that comes from knowing that they have reached out to people in need; for others, it may be the satisfaction of being knowledgable and using their skills effectively. There are probably endless numbers of ways that different therapists could describe what they get for themselves in their roles as leader.

One of the things that we as therapists, want to guard against is keeping our patients helpless or "needy". Patients tend to look to the leader for approval and direction, and it is easy to slip into a pattern of over-nurturing. What we want is for our patients to be able to find relationships outside of therapy that will be rewarding for them. While the group's initial stage may require therapists to be very directive and nurturing, the therapist should look for opportunities for patient-participants to become autonomous and self-responsible.

Kaplan talks about the striving that many therapists have to be perfect. As she emphasizes, therapist-leaders who get "hung up" with looking for perfect activities or with responding to patients in a perfect way end up wasting their own energy, and often sabotage therapy (Kaplan 1988, 124). If a therapist attempts to use the group situation to prove to him or herself that he or she is worthy, it becomes very difficult to let patients be themselves. They have to be "perfect" patients too, to prove that the therapist has done an exemplary job. Failing this, patients can end up being the target of therapists' anger and frustrations.

Therapists are just like anybody else. When they put all of their energy into one place, and their self- worth depends on one person or activity, they are more vulnerable. Being a group leader can bring many rewards. It can also be experienced as a weighty responsibility to the leader. If leaders feel worthwhile in other areas in which they work, and know people outside of work who value their contributions, it is easier for them to keep the ups and downs of the therapy experience in perspective.

Therapist as Part of the Milieu

As was stressed earlier, the individual therapist is part of the greater milieu of treatment. As such, therapists contribute as individuals; in addition, they represent the activity and profession with which they are associated. Vital is the therapist's understanding of how he or she is perceived by others in the milieu (patients, supporting and professional staff, and administration). If therapists are to possess and make use of this information, four steps are involved: (1) They need to communicate to others that they are open to feedback; (2) They need to allow this feedback to be assimilated by the self; (3) They need to realistically assess the feedback in terms of its validity; and (4) If discrepancies exist between therapist's self-image and how the therapist is seen by others, there is further work to be done.

Chapter Summary

Whether correcting discrepancies or planning a group, therapist-leaders need to have a clear sense of self and the elements which contribute to who they are personally and professionally. Personally, leaders need to be aware of their values, their views of others, their own boundaries, and the expectations they have of themselves and others. Professionally, leaders need a broad understanding of their professional roles and responsibilities, a specific understanding of their role in the therapeutic milieu and a sense of the adequacy of their knowledge and expertise.

Summary of Group Input

Before group leaders can make clinical judgments about groups — ongoing or projected — they should consider what they have to work with: the physical and emotional environment, the staff and patient population, the treatment modalities, and the leaders themselves. The system perspective attempts to consider the whole that is created when these elements come together rather than look at the elements as separate.

As we prepare to move from the discussion of group input, we could ask many questions about the "whole" of the treatment system. The following questions are offered so that you, the potential group leader have a place to begin.

1. *What is the primary mission of this treatment setting?*

   What are staff and non-treatment personnel trying to accomplish. Answers may include: a) the identification of the primary patient problems handled and possible treatment goals, b) the understanding of how this particular program contributes to the larger community and health delivery system and c) the achievement of nontreatment goals related to education, research, and provision of living alternatives for those patients no longer seen as treatable.

2. *How does it "feel" for patients and for staff to function within this setting or program?*

   While some could refer to this as the emotional climate, it goes beyond emotions. For staff and support personnel satisfaction within a treatment setting will be influenced by a) the expectations that they have for themselves that they can (or can't) succeed in achieving rewarding and growth producing experiences, b) the existence of beliefs about control and power; feelings about their ability to behave in accordance with their own beliefs and values, and c) practical matters such as those related to pay, benefits, scheduling, and comfortable physical surroundings.

   It is often very instructive to ask patients how the setting "feels" to them. Frequently staff who think they have everything under control will discover that patients are very aware of anxiety, anger or discontent in the staff. Patients can benefit from flourishing positive energy, optimism, and belief in the efficacy of treatment.

3. *What are the values and goals shared by other care providers, those of service and nonservice personnel who make up the treatment milieu? Are they compatible with my philosophies, values, and goals?*

It is not that everyone needs to think identically. However, there are certain core goals and values that need to be shared if everyone is to be "pulling" in the same direction. This enhances the therapist's feeling that he or she is a part of the greater system, and keeps staff from undermining what another is doing.

As therapists we can learn from ideologies that are different from our own, and can learn to work with treatment methods that are perhaps less familiar. In fact, the influx of new information and challenging concepts can help to energize all of those in the treatment milieu. However, as therapists prepare to try out their leader role and progress into the process of group treatment, they will need to find a style and theory base that fits the needs and values of the patient group, their own values and philosophies, and the philosophies and goals of the treatment setting.

4. *How does my particular activity group therapy focus fit into the overall mission of the setting?*

As therapists, we sometimes want to strike out and "do our thing," perhaps hoping to break ground for the sake of our own development or on behalf of increasing opportunities for patients. However, we need to evaluate carefully how our treatment contributes to the whole system, and not pursue our own activity interests in lieu of the needs of the larger whole.

For example, if an activity group is in progress or in the planning stage, the therapist should be able to assess if the group's goals are consistent with the mission of the treatment program.

5. *What are the methods of communication used within this treatment system?*

If a system is to function optimally, information needs to pass through the system, effecting a response as needed for system maintenance. A part of this involves the everyday sharing of ideas and information among all personnel. Institutions that rely on secret-keeping, or allow only the so-called authorities to be knowledgeable, not only discount everyone else, but also fail to appreciate the functional relatedness of a system. Sometimes breakdowns in communication are not intentional, but are the result of staff being busy, frequent personnel changes, or simply that information sharing has not been made a priority.

6. *What is the hierarchy of authority within the institution or program setting?*

There exist both formal and informal rules that determine how program decisions are made and implemented. Sometimes those persons identified as policy makers are less influential than those that are subordinate but powerful in the formal hierarchy. When organizing a new group or gaining support for changes in an existing group, it is important to know (a) to whom one need speak, and (b) what it is one need say or ask.

7. *Do others see my roles and activities as I do?*

One of the authors recently described an occupational therapy group that included an assertiveness component. The communication hit a snag when the psychologist sitting at the inservice said he felt that assertiveness groups should not be led by occupational therapists, but rather, were in the domain of psychology. That brings up the next question.

8. *Does my activity group complement and not duplicate the other areas of the treatment program?*

If there is an overlap, is it useful to the patient group? One of the ways that the author responded to the psychologist just mentioned was to stress that learning and practicing assertive behaviors was often a naturally occurring part of activity groups. The author also explained her position that it is helpful for patients to practice assertive behaviors in more than one context.

While a patient might use the occupational therapy activity group as a place to practice asking for assistance with tasks, or role-play bringing back a tainted steak to the grocery store, the psychologist would more appropriately work with patients on intra-family or couple issues related to assertiveness.

Team meetings are one place where different staff members can compare notes on the kinds of activities they have planned and look for ways that each can support the other.

9. *Am I clear about the kind of participation that I'd like from other treatment staff?*

Staff members, too, need ways to be active and organized, and if unfamiliar with what goes on in an activity group they may be at a total loss as to how to participate. Those coming from a verbal-psychotherapy model, for instance, might use activity group time to engage a patient in one-to-one conversation when participation in the activity was what the leader desired of them. It is up to the leader to let other staff know how they can be most helpful within the activity group.

As stated previously, these nine questions are a few of the many questions posed to gain an understanding of the group input. The authors encourage you to add to these as you work within the context of your own treatment setting.

Next we move to the elements that influence the interactions of the patient, therapist, therapeutic activity and environment — the throughput of the group system.

6
Throughput: The Group as a System of Change

Focus Questions

1. What factors contribute to group cohesion?
2. What factors influence a patient's desire to join a group?
3. How can the therapist help to create a physically and emotionally safe treatment group environment?
4. What is meant by empowering a patient?
5. What is the 'here and now' of a group?

In this and the next several chapters, we turn our attention to the internal workings of the group. In system language, this is the group's throughput. Throughput can be thought of as "where the action is", and much of our discussion later in the book will be directed towards the facilitation of group action. These chapters are also about something perhaps more basic: What makes a group a "group," and how does a therapeutic group facilitate therapeutic change?

What is a Group?

The activity, elements of the environment, patients, and the therapist-leader come together, and one assumes, a group is born. But is it always? Groups have been defined in many ways, both within and outside of therapy literature. Some definitions stress that members share something in common, a common goal (Brilhart 1978; Shaw 1982; Yalom 1970; Mosey 1973); some stress member interdependence (Cartwright 1968; Lewin 1951; Shaw 1974); others stress perception of the group as a distinct entity either by the members or by outsiders (Shaw 1981; Knowles and Knowles 1959). Earlier, the therapeutic group was described as a system of relationships that facilitates member change. We can here expand upon that definition, with the understanding that this text is especially concerned with change as it relates to the ability of group members to be active, organized and effectively boundaried. These five additional characteristics were articulated by Brilhart (1978, 20-21) and are cited also by Fisher (1980, 17). A group is a system of relationships in which:

1. The number of people is sufficiently small for each to be aware of and have some reaction to each other;

2. Members have mutually interdependent purpose;

3. Each person has a sense of belonging to the group;

4. There exists oral interaction (or an opportunity for it, in that there is sufficient face-to-face contact to allow for feedback and reciprocity);

5. There exist norms of behavior accepted by all members.

Those who study and/or conduct groups look at the mechanics of the group, called the group's structure. To review, *group structure* includes (1) the group's goals and rationale, (2) criteria for patient selection, (3) specifics related to group size, meeting environment, length and frequency of group sessions, and (4) organizational rules. They also look at group process. *Group process* refers to what happens once the group gets going. When people talk about group process, they often describe not only what has happened among group members but how (and sometimes why) it happened. If the result of the group experience could be equally accomplished by the therapist's treating each person separately, there would be little point to using a group format, except for the conservation of time. What is proposed is that there are therapeutic advantages to using an activity group format. We can prepare for the exploration of group structure and process by trying to answer the question, "What is necessary for a group as a system to facilitate desired change?" Holding the answers to this in mind, the therapist has a guide for creating a group structure and facilitating certain aspects of process.

Group Cohesion

First and foremost, if a group is to be optimal in its ability to facilitate change, participants in the group need to experience a sense of belonging to the group. This is referred to as group cohesion.

Group cohesion has been described as the attraction the group has for the participants and the attraction participants have for each other (Yalom 1970, 56; Cartwright 1968; Fisher 1980; Frank 1957). In other words, members have the feeling, "I belong to the group," or "We are a group and not just a bunch of people who happen to be gathered together." This is the "sense of groupness" referred to earlier.

We feel that group cohesion should be viewed as always on a continuum, with no absolute high or low ceiling. Once several people have been brought together in one place and time, there will be some (however slight) suggestion of cohesion. On the other hand, no matter how cohesive a group seems to be, it is impossible that it could not become any more cohesive.

Factors that Influence Cohesion

Cohesion has been discussed extensively as an attribute of group process (Frank 1957; Yalom 1970; Heslin and Dunphy 1964; Cartwright 1951 and 1968; Fisher 1980; Saretsky 1977; Kellerman 1981). The following have been cited as factors that increase group cohesion: (a) members have a personal liking for each other, (b) members see similarities among themselves, (c) there is stability in group membership, (d) participants perceive that they are liked and approved of by others in the group, (e) participants see the group as meeting their personal needs, (f) the group meets frequently, (g) members feel freedom to participate, and (h) individuals in the group perceive themselves as able to effectively resolve group tensions and group problems.

In general, a group is more likely to feel like a "group" if the participants have ample opportunity to get to know each other, perceive similarities among themselves, and have a chance to problem solve together. In terms of system theory, group cohesion implies the existence of boundaries. That is, the group knows itself as separate from whatever else and whoever else exists in the larger environment. This knowledge can be used by the therapist-leader who is trying to enhance group cohesion. Unlike the open-door welcome of "Mom" that makes all the neighborhood kids feel at home, the therapist might choose to emphasize the closed nature of the group.

Short Group Life

These more general observations about group cohesion relate to some of the specific attributes of small therapeutic activity groups. The first of these relates to the length of the group.

Occupactional therapy, along with other medical and social interventions, has had to respond to mandates for shortened length of inpatient, and often outpatient care. In acute care, as discussed earlier, many instances exist in which a group meets just once, only to have a substantial change in membership. Groups that meet only once also result when therapists are called   at the last moment to come up with something to do for scatterred, bored, or "needy" patients This short-term activity group does not beget anywhere near the level of group cohesion that is optimally found.

One can ask then, how reasonable is it to expect that patients will experience group identification or the quality of relationships that enable problem resolution? Is group cohesion an untenable goal in one-time or very short-term activity groups? Yes and no. If one sees cohesion as a continuum, then one would have a low expectation for cohesion in groups that have a short life. That needn't mean that no group identity or system of relationships could evolve. It's not different conceptually than what happens in a brief one-to-one relationship. If you, as a therapist, work with a patient only briefly, even just once, then what you and this individual hope to accomplish will be less extensive, in part because there is less time to get to know each other and less opportunity to work toward goals. But even one meeting creates some level of relationship. One goal of short-term therapy may be to increase the participant's receptivity to subsequent therapy.

Members See Similarities Among Themselves

If members are to see similarities among themselves, they have to have an opportunity to spend time together, to share thoughts and experiences.

Patients' anxiety about their own limitations and boundaries is a significant factor at work against the perception of similarities. Therapists from all specialities can undoubtedly remember patients who have insisted, "I don't want to be like them (the other group members). They are crazy (or sick, or old)." It's the case of wanting to belong to an exclusive club, only in reverse. Yalom refers to this as the "fear of contagion" (Yalom 1970, 220).

This can be viewed as a form of resistance or denial, anxiety regarding loss of personal boundaries, or an expression of patient concerns regarding safety and trust. In any case, the therapist can at times be helpful by enabling patients to clarify their present concerns. Sometimes, just getting a patient to an initial group session and giving them a chance to see that other patients really aren't so different or frightening can be useful. If patients can not overcome this move to disassociate from the group, group goals are compromised.

Goal Accomplishment and Problem Resolution

Activity groups are not necessarily more goal oriented than verbal groups. However, the attainment of some goals and problem resolution may be more evident in the visible end-product created by the group. Especially when the group's life is short, the task(s) accomplished by the group are evidence of what they have been able to do with their combined efforts, even in a short time. This should not suggest that the process oriented goals of the activity group have been abdicated. Rather, when patients have an activity to which they can relate, process skills are often made easier. For example, it is sometimes less stressful to engage in casual social conversation when working with others to assemble food baskets for the homeless than it is to make idle conversation with people sitting in the hospital dayroom.

Group Attraction

If a group is to be optimal in its influence on member change, the group must be attractive to its members. (Cartwright, 1968)

The group becomes more attractive, of course, when it is perceived as meeting member needs, and when it is viewed as relevant. One reason a group may be unattractive relates to patient fears that in a group they will receive less personal attention. Attractiveness relates also to the prestige of the group as a whole, and the prestige of those individuals in the group. We already discussed reasons why a group might seem unattractive, specifically, because its members and their ills are seen as undesirable. This impediment can occur with any kind of treatment group, and is certainly not specific to activity groups. Therapeutic activity groups do, however, have some of their own prestige problems. These can be best understood within the context of the larger systems in which therapy occurs.

Most, though not all, occupational therapy groups are carried out in a medically-oriented, health-care delivery system. Within the medical model, the physician is at the top of the hierarchy, and most often it is the physician's association with a treatment process or modality that gives it credence in the patient's eyes. Unless activity groups are being led by a physician, their value as compared to physician led groups may be questioned.

The focus within the group may raise issues related to socio-cultural values. Leisure pursuits and recreation are considered a luxury of the mid and upper classes in everyday life, but when patients see "play" being used for therapy, they often doubt the benefits and seriousness of the group experience.

Because activity groups can often accomodate adults who would not be capable of participating in verbal, insight-oriented groups (e.g. psycho-therapy group), occupational therapists are frequently asked to include less verbal and perhaps lower-functioning patients in their groups. The result in mental health care is sometimes a separation of patients into two categories; the higher level (those who attend psychotherapy) and the lower level (those who attend the activity group). Such identification is quickly surmised by even confused patients.

Finally, group attractiveness decreases when participation is not voluntary. None of us is likely to feel that we are involved in a prestigious group when it is one we are required to attend, rather than one in which we have chosen to participate.

As group leaders we can not *force* patients to view the activity group as desirable, but we are responsible for creating a group structure that is relevant to the group's needs, for facilitating a tone of respect within the group, and for educating staff and patients about the purpose, process and benefits of activity.

Here and Now

If a group is to exert optimal influence on its members, it must focus on the here-and-now.

This may not be at issue in physical medicine to the extent that it can be in mental health treatment. Both therapists and patients in mental health have some ghosts lingering from early Freudian theories where patient history was emphasized. It is instructive to note, however, that Freud himself recognized that while history might contain clues regarding behavior and feelings held in the present, it was only when patients could experience new relationships   that the goals of therapy could be accom-plished.

What the "here and now" means is that the focus of attention is on the interactions that occur among members in the group and/or the interaction between patient and activity medium during the activity proc-ess. Emphasis is placed here because that is "where the action is."

Occupational therapists may use group activities that involve reminis-cence (as in the example used earlier related to the "War of the World" tape), and other activities might evoke patient responses about "then and there" (experiences outside of the group setting). However, just as in the reminiscence group, the therapist-leader does not allow the past to stay the center of attention. Rather he or she ties the material to the present: e.g., "How does that (experience of yesterday) compare with what you are feeling right now?" or "How does that experience (at home) contrast with what has gone on in our group today?"

As tantalizing or as troublesome as past experiences outside the group might seem they are not available to the rest of the membership and cannot be changed during the group's meeting. They do not invite patient participation; rather, they place other group members in a spectator role.

Safety

If a group is to facilitate goal attainment, there must be no question that the group is a safe place to be.

If this seems a given, we propose that it can be a significant, and, unfortunately, sometimes hidden issue for both therapist and patient. *Safety* here refers to both physical and emotional safety. Ensuring safety requires knowledge, empathy and sound judgment by the therapist-leader. We can't resist the urge here to suggest that if group leaders can and will try to remember how they have felt in new, and, especially, medically related situations where *they* were the patient, they may have a much better appreciation for unspoken safety concerns.

Both physical and emotional safety depends largely on the patient having confidence that his/her welfare is of prime concern to the group leader; that the therapist is knowledegable in the areas pertinent to their problems; and that the therapist is appropriately in charge, using only accepted therapeutic techniques.

Control

Patients need to be certain, too, that they will have control in the therapy group. For instance, they need to trust that they will not be forced to do anything that they find distasteful. No one wants to be embarrassed in a group, and people have varying degrees of comfort with new behaviors or making personal matters public. If a patient chooses to take risks, he or she needs to feel that it was his or her choice, and not a result of being shamed or 'needled' into it. In systems language, they need to know that their personal boundaries are respected. Also related to boundaries is the patient's need to be apprised of what personal information can (and can not) be expected to stay private and the role of confidentiality in the group.

Predictability

Giving patients information is one way to empower them and give them control. They should know what to expect within the parameters of their treatment, what is expected of them, and why the treatment course is to follow as it has been planned. Such information makes therapy experiences more predictable. We all feel safer in situations that are at least somewhat predictable, because we have a way to organize our perceptions, prepare a response, and a means to assess the success of what has been accomplished.

Open Communication

Another vital constituent of a safe setting is the existence of open communciation. Patients need to know that they can raise questions and voice concerns and to believe that they are understood. On the flip side, they need opportunities to reach out and express their support and concern for others in the group. Therapists realize, too, that small concerns are much more likely to become destructive when individuals are encouraged to just "go along" and keep their concerns to themselves. These hidden concerns can interfere with the group process and its goals and may distract the participants from their individual goals and group tasks.

Patient Advocates

Patients do not necessarily come into therapy as wise consumers, despite the number of choices that may exist in terms of treatment alternatives. Especially when responding to physical or emotional trauma, an individual may not be capable of asking for the kind of information which would enhance their feeling of control. Even patients with many questions about their care may be too distressed initially to integrate what they've been told. Those patients who seem especially compliant, who show up at whatever therapies they've been directed to, do not necessarily feel safe and ready to start treatment either. This is an important reason for helpers to see themselves as patient advocates. *Advocacy* means that therapists strive to enable patients to make responsible, informed choices; that, when needed, they intervene on behalf of the patient to maintain the patient's welfare; that they respond compassionately to the patient; and that they strive to improve the patient's quality of life.

Therapist Safety Needs

Therapists have safety needs also. No therapist can be expected to be effective as a group leader if he or she is overly concerned that patients will hurt themselves or anyone else or be felled by a cardiac arrest. Nor do therapists do their best work when they are worried about litigation or miserable group failure. Therapist-leaders can enhance their own safety by feeling confident that they are current and knowledgable in all aspects of the therapy in which they engage. As discussed, this includes being aware of their personal and professional limitations, and knowing when to ask for staff support and when to refer patients to other therapists. Although a therapist can get caught up in feeling that he or she should be able to "do it all" that certainly is not true. In tumultuous groups, for example, a co-leader can be a wonderful source of support and may be a very necessary element in group management. If co-leaders aren't available for unpredictable groups, it makes good sense to ask for staff back-up and/or to meet in a setting that is visible to the rest of the treatment community.

Of course, any new situation (whether you're a patient or therapist) can involve fear that needs to be tolerated. This is a part of becoming familiar with a new experience. Not all anxiety can be eliminated, but creating a safe, patient-centered therapeutic experience is the basis of ethical and professional conduct. It serves as the necessary foundation for whatever else ensues in treatment. The irony is that when we as professionals know that we have done all we reasonably can to establish a safe and trustworthy environment in our group, we can feel more at ease.

A safe environment also suggests ethical practice. Group leaders are sensitive to professional ethics; they are being increasingly addresssed in the professional literature (see, for example, Lakin 1986; Laben and McLean 1984; Woody 1984; Stanley 1985). Since this space does not allow us to extensively review all the current ethical concerns, we've combined the predominant thoughts found in the literature with our own experiences to provide a list of questions that group leaders can ask to evaluate the safety factors in their group. Please refer to figure 6.1

Factors that Facilitate Change and Group Outcome

If the therapist-leader has fostered a group situation that meets the preceding criteria (the group has some level of cohesion, it focuses on the here-and-now, members feel attraction to the group, and they experience it as a safe place to be), then what Yalom refers to as the "therapeutic factors" in the group come into being. These are discussed in detail in Yalom's classic group text *The Theory and Practice of Group Psychotherapy* (1970) and summarized in his later text, *Inpatient Group Psychotherapy* (1983). These eleven factors are:

1. *Instillation of hope.* Patients at various functional levels have renewed optimism as they hear similar problems and see others take risks. Almost inevitably some patients will be demonstrating

progress in areas where others are just beginning. Seeing others succeed conveys the message, "If they can improve, so can I."

2. *Universality.* Patients meet persons with similar problems and experiences and realize that they are not unique. This can help to open up personal boundaries and decrease the individual's sense of isolation.

3. *Imparting of information.* Patients gain implicit and explicit information regarding the meaning and management of their symptoms, and feedback about their interpersonal style.

4. *Altruism.* From group interactions and interactions within the activity, patients learn that they can be helpful and contribute. This works to increase their sense of self-worth, and their belief in what they have to offer.

5. *The corrective recapitulation of the primary family group.* In the group, patients can re-experience family conflicts (or what have been for them typical social interactions) and be exposed to and try out more adaptive ways of responding.

6. *Development of specific social skills.* During the group, patients have the opportunity to listen, express empathy, and respond in other socially acceptable ways.

7. *Imitative behavior.* Patients learn from other patients and staff via role-modeling or through vicarious learning.

8. *Catharsis.* Patients can learn that it's okay to experience and express feeling, and they have an opportunity to do so in the group.

9. *Existential factors.* In the group, patients can work through concerns regarding death, freedom, isolation, meaninglessness, and other concerns common to all persons. Further, they come to grips with their own responsibility within the group.

10. *Cohesiveness.* The patients in the group develop a sense of belonging to the group and feel valued by others.

11. *Interpersonal learning.* In a here-and-now social microcosm, patients learn that how they behave in the group is similar to how they behave in their social milieu.

It is emphasized that these factors relate to the group-as-a-system, and not to the activity, per se. In the group system they help participants achieve their individual goals and support the group process that maintains the group structure. They can also influence other aspects of the group outcome, because they facilitate feedback and can influence the process of termination.

**Ensuring Group Safety:
A Checklist for the Therapist**

---

1. Am I working only within my area of expertise?
2. Do I have the necessary credentials, and are patients aware of my credentials?
3. Do I have a screening process to determine the patient's group readiness?
4. Does each member know his or her own and the group's goals? Are the two compatible?
5. Have I been careful not to promise (even by implication) more than I am able to achieve?
6. Does each participant know how goal attainment will be evaluated?
7. What have I done to ensure patient confidentiality?
8. Do patients understand the concept of confidentiality?
9. Do I have a system of clear and accurate record keeping?
10. Are other staff well informed about what occurs during my group?
11. Do I have the degree of control within my group that is needed by the group?
12. If a patient or patients become unmanageable, who do I have available to assist?
13. What physical and emotional risks are there in the techniques, tools or activities used in the group?
14. What limits, rules and other boundaries ensure adequate safety?
15. Do I have an accurate inventory of tools and supplies? Would I know if something was missing?
16. Do I scrupulously avoid sexually suggestive contact?
17. Does each patient understand the financial expense of of the group and know who is expected to pay?
18. Does the group's atmosphere encourage patients to voice any concerns they might be having?
19. What norms of behavior have been established in the group that convey respect for the individual's right to privacy? to emotional boundaries? for other personal needs?
20. Do I feel comfortable to refer patients outside my skill area?

Figure 6.1   Ensuring Group Safety

Chapter Summary

In this chapter we have attempted to make explicit some commonly held beliefs about what is needed for a group to succeed and be a therapeutic experience. Despite what research and our own experiences tell us about group cohesion and the therapeutic influences at work in a group, there are still many unknowns. We've probably all been in situations where a well-planned group just didn't "gel". Therapists can put a good deal of energy into doing the "correct" things with a patient group, only to have the group fall flat.

Although the leader can not control the group outcome he or she can reflect on the experience and ask questions. This process, sometimes referred to as clinical reasoning begins not with answers, but with having an idea of the kind of questions to ask.

If you as reader find yourself leading or participating in a group that is not coming together as hoped, we propose asking questions such as those that follow. (Student readers, try to reflect on classroom or fieldwork groups in which you participate.) If you're a person who prefers answers over questions, be assured that in chapters 9 and 10, we will provide some ideas and suggestions that can be used to help mobilize a group and facilitate the group process.

Cohesion

- Do members act as if they belong to this group?

- Are they given an opportunity to express that they like each other or have similar interests?

- Are the differences between members so great that they are having a problem sensing similarities?

- What similarities do exist? How could they be amplified?

- Have members had a chance to work through problems or difficulties?

- Do members meet often enough and in a space that helps them to identify themselves as a group?

- If members are very diverse or especially needy, would it make sense to divide the group?

Group Attraction

- Does the activity group have esteem within the milieu setting?

- If there's a problem: Is the activity appropriate to the needs of the patient group? Would staff education be helpful? Are there socio-cultural barriers?

- Is participation in the group voluntary/mandatory?

Here-and-Now

- Does the group focus on events occuring within it?
- As leader, do I or does the designated leader help point out that what goes on in the group is tied to what patients need to learn in their everyday life?

Safety

- Is the group physically and emotionally a safe place to be?
- Do both patients and leader have an appropriate sense of personal control within the group?
- Do patients and leader know what to expect in the group?
- Do patients and leader feel free to raise concerns as they arise in the group?
- Is support and encouragement given freely in the group?

Other Therapeutic Factors

- Does group activity engender optimism about problem resolution and individual goal attainment?
- Do group members practice adaptive social skills?
- What do participants "get" in this group that they do not and/or could not gain elsewhere?
- What is the quality of the role modeling that occurs in the group?
- Are there indications that the group is pulling together and feeling a sense of groupness?
- As an observer, what changes have you seen in the group? Within individual members? Within yourself?

7
Throughput: Structuring the Group

Focus Questions

1. What contributes to a group's rationale?
2. What distinguishes a sound therapeutic objective?
3. How are boundaries established in a group?
4. Describe the advantages of open versus closed group membership?
5. In what ways might daily changes in the treatment milieu effect decisions about the group on a given day? Can you give examples?

Planning an activity group is described by Howe and Schwartzberg (1986, 140) as the creation of a "cognitive strategy" for intervention by the leader. The group structure, also referred to as the group's protocol (Fidler, 1969), depends on an accurate characterization of the patient group and milieu in which treatment occurs. From a system perspective, the group structure sets limits on the scope of the group and thereby contributes to the group's boundaries. The structure includes statements related to the group's: (a) purpose or rationale, (b) specific goals, (c) criteria for patient selection, (d) plan for patient preparation, (e) activities to be used, (f) other group boundaries (including group size, meeting schedule, length of sessions), (g) session format, (h) environment, (i) special strategies that may be indicated, including those related to leadership, process, and safety, and (j) expected outcome.

Setting up the activity group involves gathering ample information and making many choices. While it would be nice to conceptualize this process as a neat package of unalterable steps; frequently, many steps are taken simultaneously, and mutually interdependent decisions are made about interdependent systems.

The Patient as "Center"

The therapist-leader has one center, and if he or she bears that in mind, the decision-making process flows more smoothly. The 'center' is the patient (or patients). Every decision that is made about how to structure the group and the environment, how to lead the group, and other practical concerns always returns to the question, "Does the structure that I am creating meet the identified needs and abilities of my patient group?" With this in mind, we can look at the kinds of decisions that must be made when organizing an activity group. Here this is discussed under the assumption that a new group is being formed; however that may not be the typical situation.

In most instances, therapists work in ongoing groups that respond to changing patient populations. Thus, the process of structuring the group becomes one of constantly reassessing what the patient group needs and where it is headed. There are instances where the therapist has a particular therapeutic activity he or she would like to use and then selects a patient population that could profit from it. But even then, the patients can't be expected to restructure themselves beyond their abilities to meet the group's demands. Again, it is the patient group that centers the decision making process.

Characterizing the Patient Group as a System

The therapist planning a therapeutic activity group has several kinds of assessments occurring simultaneously. On the one hand, he or she assesses the individual patient, and his/her particular therapy needs. On the other hand, the therapist is considering the larger patient group within the therapeutic milieu, and anticipating how the group might be expected to function together.

If one were a new therapist in a treatment setting, one would form some initial impressions about the treatment setting and the patients:

- What kind of people come to this center?
- What are they coming for?
- What is this center best known for?
- What are some common themes in the patients' histories?
- Where are most patients expected to go after treatment?
- How long is one be expected to stay in treatment?

This initial characterization is not born only from reading histories and talking to staff (although that will give one some information); but from the formation of a personal impression, based on professional knowledge–the kind one gains from being with the patient group without a formal assessment in hand, and talking or spending quiet time with the group.

Also, the therapist-leader recognizes that a group of patients will change daily, in some ways, depending on what has happened in the treatment milieu and in each person's own life. The therapist asks him or herself:

- What are the current pressing issues at this treatment center?
- Are there any current crises?
- Are there staff changes?
- Are there favorite patients that have left or are leaving?
- Does the group seem especially fretful or optimistic?
- What is the emotional tone of the day?

There are several possible tools the therapist might use to help conceptualize the group as a whole system. The Milieu Assessment introduced earlier (fig. 3.4) may be useful for this. The therapist might also try to do one or more of the following:

1. Give three words that characterize most of the individuals in the group;
2. Give one to three common concerns held by all the group members;
3. Assume that you are speaking to a stranger and describe the treatment center in three sentences or less.

As much as you might know about each patient, try to step back from the details, and get a feel for the place and the group as a whole.

Establishing the Activity Group's Rationale

Posed as questions, the therapist-leader is asking, "Given what I know about *this* group of patients, within the boundaries set by this treatment center, what can I realistically hope to accomplish with the participants in an activity group? What will be the group's goals?"

Realistic Aims

As stressed by Yalom, the group cannot be expected to cure everything that is problematic in the patient's life (Yalom 1970). The leader needs to understand the roles played by other interventions, medications, and available treatment modalities. The therapist must also have a realistic idea of what problems are remediable, and what the patient must learn to accept. For example, it is not reasonable to expect that a group activity will "cure" psychosis, or eliminate organic brain changes. However, the activity group might help the impaired patient to become more aware of the environment and others' expectations for behavior, and it can give the patient a safe place to learn and practice more adaptive behaviors. In geriatric care, the activity group should not be expected to eliminate loneliness or replace family members' visits. However, it can provide stimulation and a vehicle for the exploration and validation of feelings. And, in physical rehabilitation, the group can't eliminate paralysis in patients with spinal cord lesions. Rather, the group is a place for patients to learn adaptive skills while being given support by others who have similar feelings or frustrations. In all of these, participation in activities can contribute to an improved quality of life.

The Larger Framework

A significant contributor to the group's rationale is the therapist-leader's theoretical frame of reference; i.e., the therapist's organization of information related to function and dysfunction, the therapist's conception of treatment priorities, and the use of an identified activity to achieve these.

For example, when a therapist designs a group around the concept of improving one's self-image, the leader may use a creative or expressive activity to increase insight into one's image through a self-image collage–a projective/insightful approach. Or the therapist might seek to improve the patient's self-image through a group that teaches personal hygiene skills or a weight reduction program; an educational/skill development approach. The therapist may design a structured activity group, where a role collage and feedback discussion are used to identify the social roles that one assumes, a social network approach. The group example, Self Image Collage (see part 2 of this text) could be adapted to meet some of these treatment goals based upon varied frames of reference.

Additionally, the rationale of the activity group is related to the socio-cultural connotations of the activities that serve as the group's focus. For example, when a "work" activity is used in the group, the rationale of the group is partly shaped by the value placed on work in our culture and the resulting satisfaction gained by people when they have accomplished a work task. Groups using play and leisure activity have as part of their rationale the belief that recreation facilitates physical and emotional renewal; therefore, it is a significant contributor to a person's well-being.

Group Rationale Stated as Goals

All activity groups strive to enable their participants to be active. The life of the group depends on this. Most generally, therapeutic activity groups also have as a part of their rationale the creation of a context in which patients can give and receive constructive feedback, experience a healthy social environment that facilitates social learning, and build other specific skills related to physical, psychological, cognitive, and/or spiritual areas. When creating a group, the therapist identifies the common problems or characteristics that exist among the participants. Common characteristics will help define the group's abilities and interests, and, together with common problems, are used to identify the preliminary group objectives, also referred to as group goals. *Objectives* are statements which identify what the patient will gain or be able to do when the group is completed. These goal statements may include conditions for behavioral performance and the criteria which will be used by the therapist and patient to judge if the intended outcomes are achieved. Group objectives should be achievable and accomodate individual standards. As such, group goals are a way that the group rationale becomes articulated, specifically in relation to member needs.

Patient Centered Goals

To use an example: Let's assume a situation at the hypothetical Washington Mental Health Center. The patient population consists primarily of young men and women who have adapted only marginally throughout their lives. Many have a history of intermittant treatment experiences. Most are in transition with no specific job, education, or living-situation plans. Some individuals have physical problems related to poor nutrition habits, inadequate hygiene, and substance abuse. Some are on medication for problems with depression and withdrawl. However, as a whole, the group is not psychotic. There are other patients at the center who are considerably older and who have been brought into treatment because of highly disruptive behavior at their places of residence. These people are receiving disability benefits, are considered unable to work and are expected to return to either full or partial care living situations.

Rather than try to meet the needs of all patients within the context of one group, the therapist envisions two distinct activity groups (see figure 7.1, Patient Centered Goals). Group A will be for the younger patients who have similar basic hygiene, social skill development, self-care, and pre-vocational exploration needs. The goals of this group are to help participants gain skills needed for semi-independent to independent function in the community, with special emphasis on their learning to use non-treatment

Member Characteristics	Group Goals	One Member's Personal Goals
Group "A" Ages 19 through 36 Marginal community adaptation History of intermittant out-patient care Non-psychotic depression and withdrawl Lack of personal and vocational goals Substance abuse Poor hygiene and poor nutrition	Participants will gain skills needed to: 1. Function independently or semi-independently in the community 2. Use non-treatment community resources 3. Improve hygiene 4. Increase socialization 5. Explore prevocational resources	(Week of April 21): 1. Patient will obtain library card prior to next session. 2. Come to meeting with hair shampooed and neatly styled. 3. Share work materials with another member during the activity experience.
Group "B" Ages 50 and above In residential care Unable to work/receiving disability benefits Highly disruptive behavior at residences Intermittant psychosis	Participants will gain skills needed to: 1. Increase attentive behavior 2. Decrease destructive or bizzare behaviors 3. Increase cooperation with treatment staff 4. Increase amount of time spent in low-demand activity	(Week of April 21) 1. Stay seated at least ten minutes during orientation portion of meeting 2. Ask politely to leave the meeting if unable to sustain group activity

Figure 7.1 Patient-Centered Goals

resources for education, employment, and leisure. Group B will be designed for those who are not expected to function without significant caretaking. The goals of this second group will be to increase attentive and appropriate behavior, to decrease bizarre or destructive behaviors, to provide information and improve medication compliance, and to provide low-demand activities to help participants to experience a sense of accomplishment and improved quality of life.

Group Centered Goals

The specificity of group goals will depend on the nature of the group and the personal style of the leader who formulates them. Clear group goals can increase the effectiveness of the group as well as facilitate the group's development and process. Effectiveness is increased when goals are understood by participants, when they provide general guidelines within which a participant can create a related personal goal or objective, when they are realistic and clearly achievable, and when group members are able to identify the benefits of the goal. (Bertcher and Maple 1977) However, group goals should also be specific enough that the group leader and those outside of the group have a means to judge whether goals are being accomplished (or, in retrospect, have been accomplished).

In the latter portion of this book, we give many examples of activity groups described in the literature. The variation in goals description is due to the different ways the group goals are specified in the works cited.

Developing a Rationale

As the group leader develops a group rationale and crystalizes group goals, he or she can ask:

- What is the purpose of this group?
- How do I expect patients to benefit?
- Why do I feel that there is a need for this kind of group?
- How does this group fit with other available treatments?
- Are the group goals specific enough that they make the group's rationale clear?
- Can group members create personal, meaningful and achievable goals for themselves within the group's goals?

- Are the group goals stated in such a way that they can guide me and others in an evaluation of the group and facilitate group modification?

- When will group goals be re-assessed?

After considering individual needs, establishing the group's goals, and developing the group rationale, participants can be selected.

Member Selection and Preparation

The selection and preparation of prospective group members can be thought of as a refinement of the process begun in the first step. In many instances, the selection and preparation processes are occurring simultaneously, so we have chosen to discuss them that way.

In some cases, the therapist will be solely in charge of determining who will or will not be in a specified activity group. In these instances, the therapist-leader uses information gathered from informal observation and dialogue, patient records, specific assessment tools, and sometimes from allowing the new member a trial run in one group meeting to determine the patient's readiness for the ongoing (or projected) group experience. If the individual is not ready to handle the demands of the group, he or she could engage in preparatory activities designed to enable eventual group involvement. Sometimes patients need time for medications to take effect to control symptoms so that they can tolerate group stimulation. While waiting for patients to stabilize, therapists can see patients individually or in pairs to establish rapport, build trust, and build their attention span. Recreation activities (e.g. going for walks and, engaging in non-competitive games, movement, and gross motor activities), casual social interactions, and allowing patients to help around the nursing unit (e.g., put away snacks, make coffee) can support patient orientation and organization. By stating clearly the criteria for member selection, the therapist allows other staff to make appropriate referrals to the group.

Homogeneity

Patient group homogeneity is frequently addressed in the discussion of patient selection. In our estimation, the benefits of a homogenous group do not necessarily outweigh those of a group whose members are very different. We all know from our own experiences that encountering individuals different from ourselves can be enriching and stimulating. It can certainly be argued that we all need to learn to understand and get along with people that are different from ourselves. Yet, if people are too different, we may find that we can't relate to them. In a group, cohesion may suffer from the lack of similarities members perceive among themselves.

Because of the demands made by the activity, itself some homogeneity may be desirable: the participants' ability to be active, organized, and effectively boundaried. Some groups are specifically aimed at participants who are at a similar functional level (see for example, the Body - Ego Movement Group and the Wheelchair Mobility Group in part 2 of this book.) However, studies in the area of behavioral learning and modeling suggest that in some cases therapists should reconsider the traditional grouping of patients by functional level. These discussions propose that lower-level patients can benefit when they are paired with higher functioning individuals with whom they can identify and who they can imitate (Perry and Bussey 1984).

In relation to the selection or screening process, the therapist-leader considers:

- What is the individual's expected length of treatment or care?

- What minimum (and perhaps maximum) abilities (active, organized, boundaried) does the prospective participant need to benefit from the activity group experience?

- Are their other specific skill requirements? For example, need the participant be able to read? To be verbal? To be able to use public transportation?

- Are there specific assessment batteries or screening procedures I wish to use in pre-group assessment?

- Need there be homogeneity related to such factors as age span, gender, physical mobility, endurance, freedom of movement within the care facility (e.g. having off-ground privileges), other?

Preparing Members

New group members are often somewhat prepared for the group during the screening process. While the therapist is learning about the new patient and ascertaining his or her therapy needs, he or she is letting the patient know about the group activities available and determining where his or her involvement would be most suitable. Once the group has been decided upon, the therapist can use the meeting time to explain what the group does, and what the patient can hope to accomplish by his or her involvement. This discussion provides an important opportunity for the patient to ask questions and express concerns, and it is especially vital that the therapist help establish a tone of open communication, concern, and empathy. The patient who is not given an opportunity to express his or her concerns early on is often the one who later displays confused or resistive group behavior.

This is also a time to establish a formal (written) or informal contract between the patient and the therapist that spells out what the patient will work towards in the group, when and how his or her progress will be evaluated, and what he or she can expect from the therapist. This is also when patients can be informed and have an opportunity to ask any questions they might have regarding attendance, confidentiality, and special group rules.

As the therapist-leader considers his/her preparation of prospective group members, the therapist can ask him or herself:

- Does the patient know what he or she is working towards in the group? Does he or she see how individual goals fit with group goals?

- Does the patient understand the requirements related to attendance, punctuality, and staying with the group?

- Does the patient understand the principle of confidentiality?

- Is the patient prepared in terms of understanding the nature of the other patients he or she can expect to encounter in the group?

- Is the patient emotionally ready to be with others in a social setting?

- Does the patient have an idea of what he or she can expect from the therapist in the group context?

- Has some level of trust and understanding between patient and therapist-leader been established?

- Has a tone been set with patients that encourages each to ask questions and reach out as needed within the group?

Answers to these questions help define the rationale and boundaries of the group and its membership. The therapist then considers which activity will facilitate accomplishment of group goals.

Selection of Activities

When the group leader selects a group activity, the therapist considers whether the group topic and activity will be relevant to the group members. Activities and topics which appeal to the members' interests, values, and needs when in the group, as well as when at home or participating in the community, are more likely to increase the members' involvment in the group experience.

The therapist may choose to determine the relevance of the activity or may seek group member opinion. In physical medicine it might be that all group participants have similar physical limitations and needs related to the physiological system. However, determining the work, social, and living priorities of participants can help the therapist introduce physical demands within the context around which members share mutual concerns. Doing this as an early group activity helps members to become more aware of their similarities.

Opinions may be surveyed through a check list of discussion topics and activity choices, assessments of physical needs, or solicitation of verbal

---

Group Member Survey

Please read each topic that has been selected for a potential group meeting. Indicate your view of the topic's importance to improving your or others' performance in a work environment by circling the number that best conveys your opinion.

3 = very important, 2 = some importance, 1 = little importance

Being assertive	3	2	1
Handling problems & complaints	3	2	1
Listening to directions	3	2	1
Projecting a professional image	3	2	1
Remembering names	3	2	1

Adapted from Carlisle, K., and Murphy, S. (1986) *Practical Motivation Handbook*. (New York: John Wiley & Sons) 24.

Figure 7.2 Group Member Survey

opinion. Figure 7.2 is a sample of a group member survey. This particular survey is used to assess the importance of specific group topics and their applicability in the work environment. Based upon group member opinion, the leader then designs learning activities which relate to group topics and can build competent work behaviors.

While member priorities won't always be solicited this formally, it is important to remember that when patients are given a say in choosing activities, it helps empower them and helps them regain self-confidence. It is a means for the therapist to do "with" and not "to" patients. In chapter 8, we discuss in more detail strategies that can be used to involve patients in decision-making.

Therapeutic paramenters of activity were addressed earlier and that discussion will not be repeated.

Here we emphasize that when activities are to be used in a group context they are also selected in accordance with their ability to promote group cohesion and development. As such, activities selected should be those that:

- Encourage member participation, as opposed to member observation
- Facilitate member feedback and validation
- Promote member interdependence and if possible give members a chance to work together to solve problems
- Focus on the here-and-now
- Provide the boundaries, level of support, and level of demand that fit with participant skills and needs.

Establishing Additional Group Boundaries

There are certain mechanics to be decided in carrying out the treatment group. With the patient and activity selection these mechanics contribute to the boundaries of the activity group, and include decisions related to: (1) group size, (2) group schedule (day, time slot, frequency, and for a total of how many sessions), (3) length of each activity session, and (4) whether the group will be open or closed to new members.

Group Size

This book is focused on the small group, which has been defined as typically but not invariably having from five to ten participants.

The therapist selecting specific group activities will need to keep the projected number of participants in mind and be aware, for example, if the activity being chosen necessitates a minimum (or maximum) number of members, or for some reason requires that the group number be even or divisible by 3 or 4.

Scheduling the Group

How often the group needs to meet per week, the total number of meetings anticipated, and when the group meets will depend, of course, on the nature of the group membership, the nature of the activities and goals of the group, and the scheduling of other activities in the patient-members' lives and in the treatment milieu.

Some patient-members will be capable of adjusting to the demands of a group that meets only once or twice a week; others will need a daily meeting in order to facilitate the transfer of information or skill development. Persons with short attention spans, difficulties with concentration, or low physical endurance often have a more positive experience in group sessions that last only twenty to thirty minutes, while others can tolerate and enjoy a meeting time twice that period. Whether the group meets for a brief or lengthy period, it should be designed to be a complete and successful experience in itself.

All the decisions made about scheduling require a respect for the interdependance of the many systems that are bearing on each other. If the activity group is occuring in a treatment center, the scheduling of treatment activities typically allows for a relative balance of high versus low demand, activity and rest.

Weekend Schedules

An interesting issue is raised in relation to therapeutic activity group being scheduled for the weekend in inpatient facilities. In some institutions, most or all treatment programming is suspended for weekends to allow patients to manage unstructured time as one does at home following the typical work week. In other centers, the prevailing philosophy is that treatment needs to be on-going throughout the patient's hospitalization and therapeutic activity groups are scheduled for weekends. This issue again exemplifies a treatment decision that can only be made in concert with other staff and in accordance with the treatment institution's philosophy of care.

Consistency

Once a meeting time is selected, patients and staff need to be aware of it. A consistent time slot is not always possible, but is a goal, since consistency helps in the maintainance of boundaries. As part of the preparation process, patients should understand the consequences for failure to attend the activity session without notifying the leader, and the therapist's response to lateness.

Open or Closed Membership

Whether working in longer or short-term treatment, the situation will arise where group members are discharged or, for other reasons, leave the group. In an open group, new patients replace those who have vacated. In the inpatient setting, this often occurs when they are admitted to the institution.

The more changes there are in membership, the more energy is needed to introduce new members. You may have been in a group where the influx of new members required the group to slow down or back-pedal as the new person was given a chance to acclimate to what the group was doing.

In some groups it doesn't make sense to allow new patients to join the group after the first or second session. With educational modules, for example, each group session may represent a step in a sequence of activities, each step necessary to the larger whole.

On going groups in which no new members enter the group are *closed groups*. A closed group doesn't suffer the disruptions of an open group, and may therefore have the advantage of group cohesion. If no new patients come into the group, however, the group size may dip lower than that desired. Also, closed groups that have been together for an extended time may become stagnant because no new ideas are being expressed.

Focusing on Group Mechanics

In summary, group mechanics contribute to the boundaries of the group. The leader planning or reviewing the group structure can ask:

Group Size

- Does the group's size fit with the activity selected and does it enable face-to-face contact and feedback among members?

- Are there sub-groupings that suggest a problem with group size?
- Did everyone who wanted to contribute to the group today have a chance to? If not, what was the reason?
- Did I as leader have a chance to respond to everyone I wanted to? If not, what was the reason?

Schedule

- What activities do patients attend before and after the activity group? Is it a good combination?
- Are other staff available to provide support if needed, or are they all busy during the group time?
- Am I seeing some consistent problems with patients getting to the group on time? What's the reason?
- Do patient behaviors indicate that the group length might be too long, not long enough, or about right?

Open or Closed

- Do I have a workable means to bring new members into the group?
- Is it reasonable to keep the group closed?
- Is anything going on that warrants re-examining the current policy related to open versus closed membership?

Group Session Format

As part of planning for the ongoing group, the therapist-leader often has in mind a general format that each group session will follow. If, for example, it is to be a reminiscence group, the leader might envision each session having one activity as its focus that can be completed in 20 to 25 minutes, chosen for its ability to stimulate remembering. The leader might also plan for a brief warm-up, such as a review of the participants' week, and a closure that encorporates the use of music from days gone by. Not every therapist who embarks on leading an ongoing group has every session's plan irrevocably set. However, leader preparations before each group session help keep the group on a therapeutic course. By allowing for flexibility and potential changes in the session's plan, the leader is able to respond to day-to-day changes in the groups needs and treatment environment. It is this flexibility that allows the group-as-a-system to function as an adaptive, open system. It is in the individual group activity session that the therapist sees clearly demonstrated the relationship of group structure to group process. For this reason, we discuss the individual session in more detail in the next chapter, which focuses on group process.

Selecting and Establishing an Environmental Setting

Realistically, the therapist-leader must have an idea of the kind of setting(s) that are available before he or she makes any definite plans for the group's activities. Ideally, the leader will be able to plan the activities that he or she feels will be most beneficial to the group, and will be able to find a suitable place to have the group meet within the institution's resource of space. We have already discussed the need for the environment to fit the demands of the activities and to provide the level of boundaries, support, and safety that is needed by the patient group. In addition, the environment should have comfortable temperature, seating and lighting; as much as possible, it should be designed to eliminate unnecessary distractions.

Specific Process Strategies

The last broad category of planning relates to defining those strategies that the leader might wish to employ to enhance group safety, task development, and group process. This includes the leader's determination of the role he or she will take within the individual group sessions, and may involve a selection of specific action-oriented techniques that are used to mobilize activity, influence member behavior, facilitate intermember feedback, enhance problem resolution, enhance task-performance, and/or improve cognitive retention and understanding. These are explored in the next chapter.

Chapter Summary

When planning a treatment activity group the therapist establishes the boundaries of the group by defining the group's structure. Group boundaries include: its rationale, group goals, the profile used to guide patient referral, the group format, the group setting, and the activity resources. When decision making, putting the patient at the center allows the therapist to plan a group that has realistic and relevant treatment goals for the individual patient, as well as the group as a whole.

8

Throughput: Group Process as a System of Events and a System for Understanding

Focus Question

1. What is meant by group process?

2. What are the main stages of group development seen in activity groups? What occurs in each stage?

3. How can group norms and roles influence the patients' participation in the group?

4. How does the group leader style influence group process and the group outcome?

5. What does the leader observe during the therapeutic activity group? How are these observations used?

Defining Group Process

Group process unfolds when all of the elements of the small group are brought together in therapeutic activity.

In a therapeutic activity group, process dimensions include (a) phases of group development; (b) the relationship of activity, verbal, and social functions; (c) communication patterns within the group, including verbal as well as action-oriented communication; (d) the mobilization and expenditure of energy; (e) management of group roles; (f) standards of behavior and how they are promoted; and (g) leader styles and the strategies used by the leader in relation to all of the preceding.

Above all, group process epitomizes the 'openness' of the system. When group process is moving optimally, it is responsive to changes in the group's needs as well as changes within those systems with which the group interacts.

Phases of Group Development

Many writers have proposed the existence of identifiable phases in the group's developmental process. While citing similar kinds of changes, these writers organize their conclusions so as to suggest three, four, or five major phases. It must be pointed out that some theorists who refer to developmental phases are referring to phases within one group session, while others are referring to phases in the group's life over many meetings. In our experience, however many phases there are, the pattern can be discerned within individual sessions as well as in the overall history of the group. We also recognize that, depending on their particular theoretical bias and professional expertise, some writers stress the emotional changes that characterize group process stages; others, emphasize changes in how the group accomplishes a specified task.

William Schutz (1960, 1967, 1971, 1973) has written about the emotional issues with which group participants must grapple during the stages of group development. He chooses the terms *inclusion, control,* and *affection* to describe the predominant emotional theme present in his three identified group phases (see Figure 8.1).

Tuckman (1965) proposes a four-phase model that describes how group process develops as a task group gets its task accomplished. The phases he cites are not based on his observation of groups, but are a synthesis of what he found in published observations. Tuckman sees group process as moving toward the resolution of two kinds of problems: social problems and task problems (Fisher 1980, 140). His four phases of group development which he terms *forming, storming, norming,* and *performing* are summarized briefly in figure 8.2.

Here we direct our discussion to the stages of group process as they tend to emerge within one group activity session. Our bias, as we have presented it throughout the book, is to see emotional, social and task issues as interdependent and inseparable within the group's process. We view models such as those of Schutz and Tuckman as useful in so far as they draw one's attention to the kinds of rhythms that occur in the individual session and the ongoing group. But, we realize that not every session can be tied neatly into any of these theoretical packages. Just as people as individuals do not go through their own development in a straight line neither do groups of persons.

Staying with a system's perspective and using our own experience, we conceptualize three major phases in the group's process. We find that three stages can be used to represent the way activity is used in a majority of our own activity groups and, more specifically, the way energy is managed within the group session.

Phase	Predominant Issues	Phase Characteristics
Phase 1: Inclusion	Will I be in or out of the group? What will be my commitment to the group?	Small talk Watching other members Getting to know members in a superficial way
Phase 2: Control	Who will be in charge? How will power be distributed in the group?	Struggles for leadership and approval Competition Disagreements
Phase 3: Affection	Will I be emotionally close or distant? Do members in the group like me, or I them?	Behavior displayed connotes positive or negative feeling Heightened emotional reactions Pairing

Figure 8.1   A Three-Phase Model of Group Development. Summarized and adapted from information in Schutz W (1973) *Elements of Encounter: A Bodymind Approach* California, Joy Press.

Phase	Referred to As	Described As
Phase 1	Forming Orientation Dependence or Inclusion phase	A period during which group members are tentative with each other; trying to establish a basic social relationship and beginning to learn about each other. In this phase, participants may ask questions about each other and the group's purpose.
Phase 2	Storming Conflict or Interdependence phase	A period during which the group begins to work on ideas and procedures for getting its job done. The group realizes the time for small talk is past and it needs to move to its central task. Conflict may emerge as members vie for power and status within the group.
Phase 3	Norming Emergence Harmony or Focused Work phase	The period in which group cohesion becomes more evident The group settles down to work. Dissent is dissipated for the sake of group unity.
Phase 4	Performing Reinforcement or Productivity phase	The period in which the group not only performs optimally but also recognizes its own success. Members tend to 'pat each other on the back' for doing a good job. Even if some participants are not fully satisfied, participants recognize that the group is coming to a close and they generally have a need to leave the group feeling it was a worthwhile experience.

Figure 8.2   A Four-Phase Model of Group Development. Summarized from Tubbs (1984) A System Approach to Small Group Interaction. Reflects the work of Tuckman (1965); Fisher (1980); Thelen and Dickerman (1949); and Bennis and Sheppard (1956, 1961).

The activity group can be conceived as having three main stages, each using energy in a different way. These stages we call the (a) preparation phase, (b) focus activity, and (c) group wrap-up/closure.

Preparation

In the preparation stage, the leader is trying to get the group on one energy wave length. For example, persons coming into the group with excess energy are given a chance to settle down, while persons coming in with very low energy will have their interest piqued, and thus be energized for further involvement. The preparatory phase is also when patients are given the information they need to internally organize the experiences that follow. Preparation can include any of the following:

a) The introduction of new members;

b) A statement or re-statement of the group's goals, either by the leader or an experienced group member;

c) A review of individual member goals;

d) A review of group norms or rules. One might, for example, emphasize the importance of confidentiality or the principle of taking turns;

e) An explanation regarding the activity to follow;

f) A didactic or lecturette component; and

g) Warm up experiences. Warm-up can include anything from casual conversation to structured exercises. An important function served by warm-up activities is that they allow patients to make a transition from their experiences before coming to the group. If they are coming from a hectic (high energy) ward milieu, they may need a chance to vent their concerns before turning their attention to something new. If coming from a low-energy pregroup situation, the warm-up can help "rev up" the group.

Focus Activity

The focus activity typically makes the greatest demand on involvement and energy. Frequently, there is one main activity or series of related activities that is central in the group's purpose. For instance, the group has come together to plan a party, or to develop a job-goals list, to play a game, or to share poetry. However, there are times when the entire group session is spent on several, more diverse activities. Ross and Burdick (1981) for example, selected several very brief activities, each of which is designed to address a different aspect of sensory-neurological function in a regressed-adult group. Even with their use of multiple activities, the reader can discern in their group descriptions the build-up, maintenance and winding down of energy that we suggest here. If using many activities in one group session the therapist need be aware that it may be more difficult for patients to develop a sense of the group's purpose and/or to internally organize their experiences in the group.

Wrap Up

Like the end of a satisfying novel, the wrap-up is the group's denouement. It represents a gradual decrease in energy level and demand. The wrap-up gives participants an opportunity to pull their thoughts together, gives them a chance to look back at what they have accomplished, and allows them time to give feedback and support to each other. We've probably all been in groups that have ended when the leader suddenly noticed the time and said, "Oops! Our time is up. It was a good group. See you next time." That type of wrap-up tends to be unsatisfying and fails to give us the sense of completion we desire. It also fails to use the opportunity to bring the learning experience full-circle. Group closure can occur in several ways, including (a) a verbal insight-oriented review of the group's activities, called *processing;* (b) members giving each other member some kind of feedback; (c) a non-verbal, relaxation experience and (d) planning for the group's next meeting. In this last instance, the group wrap-up is also serving as a bridge to the next meeting, and enhances the overall sense of cohesion and continuity.

When either planning a particular group session or reviewing one that has just occurred, the leader looks at the way activities and the verbal component were used together to establish the energy rhythm just discussed. The leader asks:

- How successful was the preparation stage in creating interest, and getting the group together as needed?
- Did the activity represent a peak experience in the group?
- Did members seem satisfied at the group's closing?
- Was there an effective wind-down of energy?
- Were there any loose ends left at the closing? How could they have been "tied up?"

Behavior Standards

The phases of group development and the activities included provide one level of boundaries and guides to the group's overall process. A second and highly significant set of guides for the process is those of the norms or standards of behavior for group participants. Normative behavior standards and group members' adherence to them help to maintain the group's identity and to promote group cohesiveness, as was discussed earlier.

Group norms can be defined as standards of acceptable behavior in a group. In therapeutic activity groups they may be explicit, as when they are formally stated within behavior contracts made with individual members and reiterated to the entire group by the leader at the group's beginning. Often norms are implicit and are evidenced by the selective approval and disapproval displayed by group participants in response to given actions. Typical norms of behavior within a therapeutic activity group include those related to punctuality, confidentiality, respect for others, active participation, tolerance for others mistakes and so on.

Norms evolve from what the patient group members and the therapist-leader share as values, for example, what is perceived as "good" for the group (or "not good"); what is viewed as therapeutic; and other beliefs regarding the elements of the therapeutic group system. The norms in a therapeutic activity group may or may not fit with the norms of other groups of which patients are a part (including, for example, family and societal groups). When they do not, patient members need to understand how and why the norms in this particular group experience are different than those of other groups.

The therapist-leader, as the designated "head", has an important initial role in determining what norms of behavior constitute desired group conduct. However, when behaviors that are expected of group members are not consistent with the group members values, these behaviors can not be expected to survive.

Thus, norms "belong" to the group and not the individual (Fisher 1980, 185). Norms usually evolve and are specific to a particular group, based on the unique collective system of values brought by group members, including the therapist.

When members follow the normative standards of the group, they are said to *conform.* Such conformity is pressured by the group and generally promotes its survival. In patient groups, much of what is labeled as unhealthy, problematic, or deviant behavior is that which fails to conform to group activity therapy norms. Later in the chapter, we discuss strategies that the leader might use to respond to such "problems", but it must be recognized that neither conformity nor deviance can be viewed categorically as good or bad. At times, a group might push conformity to the extent that healthy questioning, creativity or individual preference are disallowed. At times, deviance can be assessed as a constructive reaction to a group that has settled on unproductive norms (e.g. when it becomes a group norm for members to participate only half-heartedly.)

Member Roles

Hare (1976, 131) defines *role* as the "set of expectations which group members share concerning the behavior of a person who occupies a given position in a group" (Fisher 1980, 167) One may also view roles as the norms specific to member position.

As we discussed in chapter 3, the individual may identify him or herself as having many social or vocational roles, and these serve as a background to the group. However, these roles recede as the patient now assumes two key roles that especially influence his/her group behavior. He or she takes on both a *patient role*, and an *activity group member role*. While these roles need not be in conflict, it is perhaps wise to note that what some view as acceptable patient behaviors (e.g., behaving as if ill, being cared for, and being in a dependent position) may seem contradictory to the expectation that an activity group member be active, involved, and as capable as possible. Certainly patients in both physically and psycho-socially oriented settings are often heard voicing their concern that the demands for their involvement fail to respect their role as patient.

While all therapeutic activity group members have in common a patient (or client) role and a group member role, each will further develop aspects of those roles in a style specific to his/her unique personality and preferences, as well as in response to expectations made of him/her by other members in the group. That is, each patient's interaction role is worked out within the arena of the group experience and is thereby a product of the whole group's process, or thoughput.

Interaction Roles

Many efforts have been made to categorize common group interaction roles (see figure 8.3). The goal in a therapeutic activity system is to keep the system energized, open, active, and effectively boundaried; therefore, each role a patient takes in the group can be described as either facilitating, impeding, or tangential to the group's process. Interaction roles will either have a facilitating or nonfacilitating influence on the patient's, efforts to accomplish his or her own personal treatment goals. Futher, interaction roles influence the group's outcome (or what the group ultimately accomplishes) and the manner in which members give and receive feedback from

---

Group Task Roles

Initiating-contributing — gives new ideas, suggestions for accomplishing the group goal.

Information seeking — asks for information, facts or clarification.

Opinion seeking — seeks to get information regarding the values that underlie a suggestion.

Information giving — gives facts based upon experience or authority.

Opinion giving — gives beliefs and opinions to suggest values the group could adopt.

Elaborating — expand, clarify and hypothesize outcome of the suggestions made by other group members.

Coordinating — attempts to combine ideas, to coordinate activities and to suggest relationships among ideas.

Orienting — summarizes group progress, and raises questions regarding future directions of the group

Evaluating — compares the group progress to group performance standards.

Energizing — attempts to increase group interaction and decisions.

Assisting on procedure — helps the group achieve its goals through performing routine tasks.

Recording — documents suggestions, group decisions and outcomes in order that the group can see tangible results.

Figure 8.3a   These are roles that facilitate group process by helping to keep the system open, active, and organized. Adapted from Tubbs (1984) *A Systems Approach to Small Group Interaction* (2nd, ed.) New York: Random House (Original source Benne & Sheats [1948]).

---

* Group Maintenance Roles

Encouraging - acknowledges the contributions of others by listening, praising, being tolerant and verbalizing support for the ideas, feelings and actions of others.

Harmonizing - mediates conflicts and tensions that arise among the members during the group experience.

Compromising - yields during a conflict situation to meet a person half way or can put aside ones personal needs for the betterment of the group.

Gatekeeping and expediting - monitors the group participation and facilitates communication to increase the opportunity for all to be heard and limits members who try to monopolize the group.

Setting standards or ideals - evaluates the group process and verbalizes the group's standards (rules of conduct and protocol for interaction, procedures, etc.).

Observing - monitors and records the group's process and gives feedback , in a nonjudgmental manner, to the group regarding its performance.

Following - passively participates in the group; "serves as a group audience" through listening, passive acceptance of others and the group's events.

---

* These roles especially serve the group outcome referred to as group maintenance. They may also contibute to group process by facilitating effective organization and boundarying within the group system.

Figure 8.3b   Group Maintenance Roles. Adapted from Tubbs (1984). A Systems Approach to Small Group Interaction (2nd ed.) New York: Random House (Original source Benne & Sheets [1948]) p. 249.

---

* Individual Group Roles

Aggressing - takes advantage of others, disapproves or may attack others thoughts and ideas, may take credit for the accomplishments of others and may use malicious humor.

Blocking - behavior that prevents the group progress and development (arguing, going off on tangents, rejecting ideas without adequate consideration).

Recognition seeking - attention seeking behavior (excessive talking, boasting, or assuming a superior attitude or position in the group.

Self confessing - promoting personal concerns rather than supporting the group theme or focus.

Acting the playboy - interferes with group function and detracts from the group's task by a nonchalance attitude, "goofing off" or horseplay.

Dominating - intentionally controling and manipulating others in the group through flattery, interrupting others or "pulling rank".

Help seeking - use self derrogatory statements to get attention from others; e.g. self criticism, boasting personal limitations, expressing insecurities.

Special interest pleading - predominantly speaking about one's own biases and prejudices under the guise of speaking on behalf of others (e.g. underpriviledged) at the expense of the group task.

* These roles when acted out, tend to impede group process and detract from the achievement of group (outcome) goals, including that of group maintenance.

Figure 8.3c   Individual Roles. Adapted from Tubbs (1984). A Systems Approach to Small Group Interaction (2nd ed.) New York: Random House (Original source Benne & Sheets [1948]) p. 249.

each other. If you look again at figure 8.3, you will see that we have proposed how some familiar interaction roles are likely to affect group process and/or outcome. These should not be viewed as predictive; rather, we are trying to help the reader approach the group as a "system thinker."

At times, the role taken by a group member is familiar and comfortable since it is similar to the role they have assumed in other task or social groups. Sometimes, however, members find that other group participants expect them to assume roles that are unfamiliar, uncomfortable, or even beyond their ability. The reader may, for example, be able to recollect instances in which he or she entered a group planning to be passive, only to have others continually solicit their opinions or guidance.

Discordant Roles

Role strain occurs when a group expects a member to assume a role that includes behaviors beyond which he or she is capable. *Role conflict* results when a member is asked to assume a role that is opposite or contradictory to the one the individual typically performs in other groups. (Fisher, 1980, 172)

Patients coming into a therapy group bring with them a repertoire of role related experiences from such systems as the workplace, home, community, and other treatment or care facilities. When they are asked to assume a role within the group that is inconsistent with how they see themselves or is uncomfortable to them, several scenarios may be chosen. Among these are the following:

a) The individual patient may remove him or herself from the group;

b) The individual may reassess his or her own self-perception;

c) The individual may question their perception of what is acutally consigned to the role;

d) The individual may risk discomfort and try to adapt to new role behavior (He or she may, for example, recognize that "self" can behave differently in various situations);

e) Other members of the group may modify what is expected of any patient in that role; or

f) Other members may choose someone else to fill the role.

Reader Activity

If you as reader are involved in a group experience, we ask you to see if you can identify the following, as they pertain to the relationship of norms and roles to group process.

1. Identify three values that appear to be shared by the group members.
2. Identify three or more norms of behavior that you see as vital to the life and success of the group as a whole.
3. Pick several different group participants and name or describe the role(s) they assume within the group.
4. State whether or not you see norms and roles assumed within the group as conducive to a sound functioning group process. Why or why not?

Leader Role

The leader referred to in this chapter is the therapist responsible for planning and implementing the treatment experience. Group members (patients) may assume a leadership role in the context of a particular group experience, but do not have the therapist's responsibilities as discussed in this chapter, nor do they intentionally use the strategies described later.

Here we explore two leadership functions that are understood in a way that is specific to a system perspective. These are roles the leader plays to help mobilize energy and provide a structure. We refer to this as "organizing energy".

Mobilizing Energy

As stated previously, general system theorist von Bertalanffy leans toward the ego psychologists who say that the person is motivated to use personal energy in activity because there exists an in-born human need to explore and master self and the world (von Bertalanfy 1968). Stated another way, sitting around all day is not satisfying to most people and they usually wish to find a way to alleviate boredom.

If people have an innate urge to be active and expend energy, one can ask, "What gets in the way? Where does the energy go when patients lack the energy to get involved in a group activity?"

When persons feel threatened, either physically or emotionally, they tend to use their energy to protect themselves. This often involves stiffening personal boundaries, and drawing in to the self. The reverse process can occur wherein patients under stress expend much energy in aimless or overly diverse ways (e.g., seeking guidance from too many sources).

The things that trouble patients result in other behaviors that take energy. Worry, loss of sleep, inconsistent eating habits, physical trauma, and medications can all be energy stealers. Added to that is the energy some use in trying to put up a false front. As articulated by Schutz(1973, 16): "You must expend great amounts of energy to hide your feelings, thoughts, or wishes from other people, and even more energy to keep them from yourself. To withhold secrets requires a tightened body; it requires a curtailment of spontaneity least the secrets be revealed; it requires vigilance, shallow breathing, physical exertion, and a preoccupation with your own safety."

When patients feel the need to protect their personal boundaries and block out feedback, they may feel "too drained" to participate in an activity group. It is also important to remember that while the urge to expend energy in activity may begin with an innate drive, people learn from their experiences which activities are rewarding, relevant, and deserving of time and energy. None of us is likely to expend energy in activity that fails to appeal to our interest, that doesn't offer something that is perceived as meeting personal needs for approval, survival, learning, comfort, or pleasure. Therefore a vital part of the leader's ability to mobilize energy lies in his or her skill at selecting and presenting activities in a way that fits with the developmental level of motivation, as well as the participants' interests as both change within the group's life.

There is nothing quite as deflating to a group leader as coming into a group personally energized and ready to carry out a group activity, only to encounter a listless group devoid of any apparent energy. Gruen (1979, 63) puts the burden squarely on the leader when he says that in such a situation the leader must have "surplus energy" to put into a group of patients who have depleted their usable energy by putting it into self-defeating or pathological behavior. He proposes that this energy be conveyed in the form of an informational message from the therapist that suggests, "I know that you can change and (you) have the capacity and, eventually the strength to help yourself grow." Gruen concedes, however, that this energy is hard to define. It is not just information, and goes beyond the therapist's "interest and caring." We believe that a part of what the leader wishes to convey is the message of validation, e.g. "I know you may be feeling pretty overwhelmed by what lies ahead, ... but we'll take it one step at a time." The leader who enters the group with plenty of energy can be a significant spark in getting the momentum going, especially when what is communicated is his/her untethered belief in the activity experience and the patient group. But leaders need to stay sensitive to the chasm that a patient may experience when they sense the distance between their own lack of energy and the enthusiasm they're confronted with.

Kaplan (1988) emphasizes that in working with low-energy groups, group leaders should select activities that do not require a great deal of energy, and should pace the activity downward to the level where members can participate effectively. This is, of course, consistent with the principle of structuring the group to match the abilities of the intended participants.

Organizing Energy

Even if sufficient energy exists within the group, this does not ensure the group's success.

The following interaction occurs when the leader, watching a group of enthusiastic and usually well-organized patients, notices that today they have not succeeded in getting the group off the ground.

> Leader: "I hear a lot of conversation, but it still
> appears as if the group's having trouble getting
> organized today."

> Participant: "Yeah. Nobody can agree on what we should do."

> Leader: "Well, you know I'm here as a resource, but I'm not
> going to jump in and delegate jobs. I trust you can
> get it together."

In this group, participants have the energy to be involved, but energy is going in many different directions. Because the leader believes that the members are capable of taking charge of the group, he or she has chosen to hold back from intervening. Should the group continue to flounder, the leader might choose to intervene in order to help group members determine what is getting in the way of goal-directed activity. Or, he or she might take an active role in assisting the group to select and follow through with a group activity.

The cues for determining the extent to which the leader needs to act more as a director and less as a participant or resource comes from the ability of individual members to be active, organized, and effectively boundaried, as well as from these abilities as they are demonstrated by the group as a whole.

Situational Leadership

Hersey and Blanchard (1984, 201-204) use the term *situational leadership* to describe a leader role that adapts to the readiness or "maturity" of participants in being active, organized and boundaried within the group's context. *Maturity* is defined by them as the "ability and willingness of [group participants] to take responsibility for directing their own behavior". It is acknowledged that a group or individual may be mature enough for one task or event, but not for another. That is, individuals and groups are not believed to be mature or immature in any "total sense".

According to a model of situational leadership, there is no one best style of leadership. However, Hersey and Blanchard propose that certain styles are more likely to be successful given the identified maturity level of the group.

They say a telling style of leadership is for low maturity . Low maturity from a system perspective suggests that group members are unable and unwilling to be active on their own behalf. A *telling style* is one where the leader gives clear, specific directions, selects and supervises activities, infuses energy, and provides group boundaries. This style is exemplified in the Body-Ego Movement Group or Directive Group described in part 2 of this text.

Selling is for low to moderate maturity. This leadership approach is for groups in which participants are unable but willing to take responsibility. Members lack the skills to be self-directed. The leader organizes the group, gives directions, and provides boundaries but also supports the members' enthusiasm and reinforces any behaviors that demonstrate movement toward learning necessary skills. The leader uses explanations and tries to engage participants in two-way communication. This style is called selling because when the leader is providing direction he/she is trying to get members to "buy into" desired behavior (Hersey and Blanchard, 1984, 203). The Community Cooking Group (part 2) uses this leadership style.

Participating is the style suggested for the leader in a group at moderate to high maturity. Members at this level are regarded as able but unwilling to take responsibility for initiating and following through with a group activity. Again, open communication is needed to respond to this level of maturity as the leader tries to understand (and help the group to understand) their reluctance. The leader may be supportive and non-directive. This style is called participative because both leader and members share in deciding how the group will be conducted, with the key role of the leader being to facilitate activity and communication. This leadership style is frequently seen in educational groups such as that of the Coronary Heart Disease and Daily Function Group in part 2 of this text.

A *delegating* style is appropriate for high maturity. As in our previous example, members at this level are considered to be both able and willing (or confident) to take responsibility. In this group, the leader provides little active direction and minimal support. While the leader might identify the problem or task that confronts the group, the responsibility for developing and carrying out the group activity is given to the membership. This style is frequently seen in outpatient or transitional living groups where participants hold a weekly meeting to choose and plan their weekend schedules and activities in order to learn to structure their free time and learn to use community resources.

Other Leader Roles

All of these situational styles need to be considered flexible within themselves, because groups and group members will fluctuate in their maturity level, and therapists bring their own personal style to the leadership role. With none of these styles is it suggested that the leader remove him or herself from the group or simply do nothing. (At that point the leader could be viewed as no longer a leader at all!) The term gate-keeper has been used to describe the leader's role in a group, and it is a term that fits the system perspective especially well. As gate-keeper, the leader helps regulate what is allowed to enter the system. Further, as gate-keeper he/she is able to observe the behaviors that may indicate a change in group needs or abilities and may call for a re-evaluation of the leader's role. As gate-keeper the leader also continues to promote a safe and accepting atmosphere within the group experience.

Frequently, in occupational therapy the leader chooses to be a participant as well as an observer. In so doing, the therapist-leader assumes many roles and functions simultaneously. By getting right into the action the leader can gain a better understanding of how patients experience the activity, and if necessary, make adjustments. Patients often appreciate that the therapist doesn't distance him or herself, and they will often try to emulate desired social and task behaviors in the leader.

Observation Guides for Group Leaders

When observing group interaction the therapist seeks to monitor the gestalt of the session and get a sense of the whole picture. There is no substitute for observation of the group's natural, spontaneous interaction to understand how the elements of the group system actually function in a meaningful whole. It is only with such observation that the leader can determine the appropriate style of leadership, and gather the information needed to evaluate the group's success in meeting individual member and overall group goals. Astute observation may also help the therapist-leader to identify a need for using specific strategies to deal with various stages and/or problems specific to the group.

A summary or high point of the elements and processes that the leader can observe are represented in Figure 8.4.

Observation Guidelines

1. The physical environment and emotional climate of the activity group; changes that occur as the group ensues.
2. The energy level of individual participants; emotional investment in the group; willingness to use one's abilities to produce a group outcome.
3. The boundaries of the participants; e.g., oriented, ability to establish and maintain boundaries of oneself and support those of the group.
4. Effectiveness of the leadership; the therapist's ability to mobilize the energy in the group, keep the participants active and organized, maintain group boundaries and adapt a leader style that meets group situational needs.
5. The role of the activity; activity's ability to mobilize participants' energy, maintain the group boundaries, support the leadership style and require the participants to use their skills and abilities.
6. The feedback that occurs during the group; pattern of communication among the participants, existence of a social network, degree of flexibility in which roles are assumed, the rhythm established by the group events, and the group process.
7. Energy level of the group.
8. The group's boundaries; e.g., the norms and rules of the group, the roles in the group, the therapeutic factors that exist, the group's structure, etc.
9. The group's outcome; group theme, task accomplished, feedback, method of termination or closure, unresolved issues or tasks, etc.
10. Changes in the patient, leadership, activity or environment as the group occurred.

Figure 8.4   Observation Guide

Process Intervention

After making his or her observations, the leader may see that the group needs some help getting or keeping the process going in a positive direction. Leader strategies may be directed toward facilitating verbal or action oriented participation and/or increasing member awareness and insight. We begin by looking at specific communication strategies to facilitate dialogue among group participants during the activity experience and to enhance the members' understanding of the activity experience. These strategies include traditional communication responses and question and discussion summary approaches.

Communication Responses

Although the therapist applies them in a group setting, as leader he or she can use the same communication responses as those frequently identified with one to one counseling situations. Those used include: feedback, support, confrontation, advice and suggestions, summarizing, clarification, probing and questioning, repeating, paraphrasing, highlighting, reflection, interpretation and analysis, listening, and timing. Any of these responses when used effectively can promote participant interaction and learning. Samples of these varied responses are included in the following suggested guidelines for responding to participants during an activity group. However, we don't wish to suggest that therapists follow any guides in a wooden fashion. The goal, as we see it, is to be responsive to the unique challenges of every group.

The leader listens to participants' responses and then acknowledges the opinion(s) expressed. After listening to participants' views, the leader gives feedback by acknowledging the participants' answers ("correct" or otherwise), and encourages the other participants to share additional opinions. If an incorrect (inappropriate) response is given, you as leader never belittle the group member but encourage the person to try again, or, if appropriate, elicit assistance from other members.

Many persons new to group activites are especially concerned about appearing inept in front of their peers. Group members frequently will not interact unless they are encouraged by the group leader. If participants do not have opinions or questions even when given permission to respond or inquire, sometimes an example or suggestions will help. For example, the leader states, "When I was in a group like this before, the members frequently asked" or "When I did this activity before the participants learned" or "Since the group can't decide what to do today, let's brainstorm to identify possible activities."

When listening to responses and questions, the leader pays attention to the content as well as the attitude that the person conveys, and then responds to participants. The leader may highlight key points of the comments or provide an interpretation and ask for confirmation from the participants.

Responses or questions need not be repeated unless they were not heard by the entire group. In that case, the leader might ask the group member to repeat the question or he or she may paraphrase the participant's comment. The leader should avoid restating or unnecessarily repeating the responses of others.

After a question is posed, some leaders respond with statements such as "Good question" or "I knew you were going to ask that!" When overdone, these responses become less meaningful and can detract from the focus of the discussion. However, if the patient's question is appropriate and it reflects his improved ability to function in the group, you may want to give it special recognition.

Encourage group members to respond to each other rather than direct all communication to you. If members continue to pose questions primarily to you, you may want to solicit group opinion prior to giving your own. Sometimes patients find it difficult to disagree with the "expert" (leader) in the group especially when their response follows the leader's.

When the leader responds after several other opinions have been expressed, he or she is in a position to summarize, contrast and highlight view points as well as add an opinion (or state that he or she has nothing else to add). When you answer a question, your response should be brief and focus on key concepts. If you do not know the answer or don't have an opinion, say so. No one (even group leaders) need know everything! Another productive avenue when stumped by a question, is to tell the group that you will investigate after the group closes, and get back with the information you've found.

Responses can also be used to promote problem solving. The group leader can use responses, questions or probing which will encourage the patient to reason or hypothesize about the unknown. As participants respond to each other, the leader can help the group identify the strengths and weaknesses of the response, determine the possible effectiveness of the course of action suggested, and then summarize major issues that arise. In general, the leader responds and promotes responses which are constructive, encouraging and non-demeaning. He or she promotes multiple responses rather than "yes" or "no" answers and relates the questions and the responses to the therapy goals.

Questions to Promote Participant Communication

Therapists are sometimes cautioned against using questions because they might put patients in an uncomfortable or defensive position. However, when used effectively, questions can get group members' attention, assess members' interest in the group, validate the participants' understanding of the group experience, promote interaction among group members, increase participant involvment in the group activity, and facilitate problem solving. For that reason we choose to discuss in some detail the use of questioning as a leader strategy.

Leaders may use open (broadening), closed, fill-in-the-blank, multiple, or hypothetical questions during a group. However, the literature suggests that some are more effective than others. Each is briefly reviewed here.

Types of Questions

The *fill-in-the-blank* question is illustrated when the leader begins with, "During the group today, the role play showed you that..." and allows the members to finish the statement. Group members may not notice a fill-in-the-blank question and thus will not respond to the query because they are unaware that a question is being asked. It is preferable to state, " Now that the role play is finished ask yourself, 'What did you learn from the role play that will help you when you leave the hospital?'"

When a leader uses the question in a specific context to pose a hypothetical situation, the query is called a *hypothetical question.* Hypothetical questions give a context for what is being asked. For example, "Suppose that you are at work and your employer asks you to perform a task for which you are unqualified, what do you do?" These questions can elicit facts as well as opinions.

Multiple questions can cause the participant to be confused and feel uncertain about what is being asked. As a result, participants usually answer only one of the questions, and you have to repeat the others one at a time. It is best to avoid multiple questions.

Broadening questions are used to solicit additional information beyond that previously shared by a group member. These questions may be posed to the whole group or a specific member. Sample broadening questions: "What other alternatives might work?" "What were the reasons for your choice?" "What other factors should be considered?"

An *open question* is one in which there are multiple responses; e.g. "Please describe to the group your method for solving the problem." A *closed question* requires only a "yes" or "no" or one word response. There are some group leaders who feel that questions that require a one-word response don't need to be asked.

Question Strategies

Suggested questioning strategies recommend that questions be clear and succinct, be relevant to the group experience, be specifically stated, meet the learning needs of the group (e.g., not too difficult, nor easy, nor embarrass individual members), and be appropriate for the time frame (e.g there should be adequate time to respond to questions - the leader should not pose questions when it is time for group closure or break). Occassionally this can mean giving participants a question to think about during the interim before the next meeting.

After a question is posed, the leader should pause and allow time for the participant to think of a response and then ask for a volunteer or specific person to answer. A pause can also heighten the interest of the group. Alert the group members that a question is being asked; "Please listen to the following question" or " . . . has asked the question" or "(patient's name) has a question. . . . " When group members are alerted to a question, they may listen more carefully. It can also help them organize a response. Such cueing also decreases the likelihood that a member will be embarassed by being unable to respond because he or she didn't know that a question was being asked.

In addition to these strategies, the leader can influence the group process by the manner in which he or she responds to the behavior of group participants. Behavior management strategies are summarized next.

Behavior Management

The leader may need to respond to or manage behaviors that promote group interaction or that do not fit the standards set for the group. When an individual behaves in a way that is out of step or interferes with the group process and goal attainment, it may be for one of several reasons:

a) role strain or role conflict,

b) a lack of information or understanding about the behavior expected,

c) the patient is in some way being rewarded by the group for this behavior,

d) the behavior is related to or symptomatic of the individual patient's problem(s), or

e) the behavior is symptomatic of "unhealthy" group norms.

As therapist-leaders we are all very human and may find ourselves getting angry or frustrated when responding to behavior problems. However, it is often helpful to remind ourselves that the individual may not have set out to be destructive. In fact, some behavior problems may be a reaction to an unhealthy element or process within the group experience that needs attention. When the leader's frustration seems to block his or her ability to respond in a way that respects the integrity of each member, it may be time to ask for assistance from other treatment staff in understanding or responding to behavior problems. The following are some of the behaviors that often interfere with group process. No pat remedies are intended in the responses we review.

Silence and Non-Participation

Although leaders frequently assume that silence indicates resistance, there are several other possible reasons. The non-contributing members may feel they have nothing to offer, or they may be anxious, or they may fear their contributions will fall short of what others can do. If there are many silent or apathetic members in the group, the leader may need to reconsider the nature of the group experience or question if some hidden agendas within the group are promoting a nonparticipation norm. The leader may need to reassess treatment goals or leader strategies.

There are several strategies for responding to an inactive member. A nonverbal strategy sometimes used by leaders is to make frequent eye contact with a silent or inactive member. Or, the leader may verbally inquire, "What is causing the silence in the group today?" or "What's making it hard to get involved in our activity?" The leader may also choose to speak to the reluctant person outside of the group and provide support and encouragement for participation, or he or she support the smallest effort made to contribute during the group.

In general, persons can not be forced to participate; they need to interact at their own pace. Groups may try to pressure non-involved members to participate and be successful, but in most instances the pressured person withdraws more or avoids the group. A group atmosphere of tolerance, where less-than-perfect performances are clearly appreciated, is more likely to encourage participation.

Monopolizing Activity

On the opposite end of the continuum from non-participation are those members who monopolize the conversation or activity either to manage their anxiety or satisfy a need for attention, or because they are unaware that they are monopolizing. Their contributions may relate to the activity or detract from the group purpose and theme. If they relate, the leader may acknowledge the member's contribution, but solicit the opinions and involvement of the other group members. When verbal contributions do not relate to the specific activity experience the leader thanks the participant for the contribution and then returns the focus of the discussion to the original topic. When refocusing the group the leader may have to summarize the previous discussion or restate the group goals to get the group back on target. Or, the leader may suggest that the nonrelated or distracting contribution may be a possible agenda item for a future group experience.

Hostility and Aggression

Activities and/or group discussions may also cause strong emotional reactions. When someone is angry it is usually best to let them have some distance to "cool off" before you try to help them manage their feelings or talk with them. If you fear that they will hurt someone in the group or if they are too disruptive, you may need to ask them to leave. At that point, it may be necessary to have a staff member with them to provide extra safety and support.

It is important that the individual not view leaving a punishment, and it is often helpful if you or another staff member can later talk with the individual about tools they might use to manage their anger. You might also help them identify cues that tell them they need to remove themselves physically or emotionally from a volatile situation before they lose control.

Abusive Language or Swearing

At times strong emotions are expressed through abusive language. Some therapists and group members are tolerant of swearing while others are offended. It is okay to tell group members that their language is offensive (just as it may be in other community settings) and to ask that they find another way to express their anger. Some leaders ask the group members to respond to the behavior and to say how they feel that abusive language is influencing the group process. Once this issue is resolved, the leader returns to the group topic and activity or pursues the next aspect of the group.

Tardiness

When members arrive late the leader has a choice of asking them to sit quietly, listen, and observe; asking a fellow participant to orient them to the activity in progress; or taking the time from the group experience to do so him or herself. Regardless of the choice, it is best to choose the least disruptive. Some groups have the norm that no late-comer will be allowed into that particular session.

When a series of groups are to occur, during the first meeting the leader sets the ground rules for discussion, states the importance of being on time, and asks members to notify the leader if they will be absent.

Members can call in advance (if an outpatient group) to inform the leader, or send a message with another group member.

Threats to Quit or Leave the Group

When patients ask to leave the group prematurely it may be because the patient is uncomfortable with the present group experience, that the group is not meeting the patient's needs or that the patient is not ready to make a commitment to change. Leaders can ask members why they want to leave and then also give the group members an opportunity to discuss the person's decision to quit. Some individuals threaten to leave a group because they are testing the group's reaction. They may, for example, be hoping to hear that others care about them. Therefore, if a leader emphasizes that the choice to stay or leave is ultimately theirs, the leader needs to be careful that he or she is not giving a message that suggests that no one cares what choice the individual makes.

Consistent Absence

Some of the same reasons that people leave or quit the group also apply to those who are consistently absent. The leader can encourage the person to attend and participate so that he or she benefit from the experience. The leader may also need to evaluate the appropriateness of the treatment referral or provide an alternative treatment group.

Breakdown — Crying

Group experiences can cause strong emotional responses besides anger. If possible, allow the participant to express the emotion, but not so much as to derail the group process indefinitely. The leader can encourage the members to recognize the person's sadness, be supportive, but he or she should discourage others from overreacting or trying to make the sadness go away. At times it is sufficient for a group member to sense group support. Then the person can shift attention to the activity or discussion. If a person's burst of emotion is uncontrollable, the leader (or assistant, if there is one) can offer to escort the person from the group to another room and then sit and be with them privately.

Dishonesty

Sometimes a patient may feel pressured or "pushed into a corner", which causes him or her to be dishonest. The leader can choose to discuss this privately outside of group, or can help the person see his/her discrepancies during the group. Regardless of the choice, the leader tries to confront the person with minimal embarrassment in front of his/her peers.

Skeptical Group Member

On occassion, a group member questions the purpose as well as the effectiveness, of the group. This skepticism may represent the person's lack of information or may be an expression of anger or resistance. Thus the leader has a choice of focusing on the manner of expression or the content of the complaints. Rather than becoming defensive, the leader can ask the other group members to give their opinion or to state how they feel about the interference. Group members should be given the opportunity to give feedback to the skeptical member. In addition, the leader may invite the complaining member to make suggestions on how to improve the group experience. The leader needs to listen carefully to concerns because legitimate problems may exist of which the leader has been unaware. Once the complaint or concern has been handled, the group should not be permanently side-tracked. If the individual continues to complain,you, as the leader, may ask the group member to postpone the issue for now, while inviting the person to leave and meet with you after the group is over.

Third Degree Questioning — Interrogation

As was suggested previously, it is preferable to use questions that facilitate learning and interaction rather than those likely to cause a person to become defensive. When participants begin to interrogate each other the leader can simply state that this is not the method of inquiry that is used in therapeutic activity groups.

Intellectualization

There are various viewpoints regarding the style of interaction expected from group members. Some groups discourage intellectual interactions and push for participants to relate emotionally and express their feelings. It is important to recognize that being intellectual or taking on the role of the intellectual in a group may be the role that is most familiar to the group member. To demand that he or she give up this style, especially when he or she has little experience with any other, may be unfair. Sometimes it is more reasonable for the person to be encouraged to gradually try out "new waters". The leader might, for instance, model the way "I think" statements can become "I feel" statements, and aid the participant to start by making just one or two feeling statements in a group. While concerned about the effect of intellectualization on the whole group, the leader needs to understand that change can be difficult and must begin with a personal commitment. The leader challenge is to use the patient's intellectualization or emotion to facilitate effective interaction, while allowing the patient to feel okay about him or herself and his or her participation in the activity.

Fault Finding, Blaming, Scapegoating

Sometimes when group members are disappointed in the outcome, they may blame others for the failure. The leader should try to prevent scapegoating and redirect the assault to a problem on which all group members can focus; e.g. "Paul, you suggest that Mary's refusal to work on the activity kept your team from finishing on time. Do you feel, Paul, that your team had any other alternatives which would have helped it complete the project on time?" or "Philip, you suggest that Sue is avoiding the issue. Do you feel that you react similarly under similar work circumstances?"

In general, the group leader encourages each person to take responsibility for him or herself. Those who blame others or interfere with what others are trying to do may be approached in or outside of the group.

Making Excuses — Defensive

Sometimes participants make many excuses for their behavior. When this occurs, the leader can encourage group members to give their reactions to the defensive behavior. The intent should not be to put the participant on an interminable hot-seat. It may be useful to encourge others in the group to remember times they too made excuses, and to reflect on how they were feeling. The leader might need to determine if role strain or role conflict is partially a cause for a participant's defensive posture.

Chapter Summary

The process in a therapeutic activity group tends to develop according to a rhythm that has three discernable phases. The way that energy is spent by group members is influenced by the roles and normative standards set by the group, by the amount of usable energy brought to the activity, and by the enthusiasm members have for the activity(s) presented.

The leader has many functions specific to group process. Primary among these is the encouragement and support of all group member's participation; and his or her helping members to learn from their group experiences. This leader function can be thought of as keeping the group system open and responsive. Leaders who are successful at promoting a healthy, functioning systems are most likely those persons whose intervention in the group are suited to the group's level of maturity.

In this chapter, we focused especially on the roles of dialogue within an activity group. In the next chapter, we look more closely at ways in which the therapist can facilitate patient participation in the group's activity, and enhance patient learning.

9

Throughput: Promoting Participation and Learning

Focus Questions

1. What strategies are used to structure the activity experience and facilitate the activity process?

2. How does activity processing influence group throughput and outcome?

3. What is the role of personal committment in the activity group?

4. How does group discussion influence group throughput?

The therapeutic activity is central to the group's process and outcome. However, it is not only the task itself, but also the leader's ability to use and process activities which promotes activity as a catalyst for achieving group goals, and for facilitating discussion, problem solving, skill practice and learning. This chapter describes actions which leaders can take to maximize the impact of activity upon group process. From the many strategies described in the literature, we have chosen the following: brainstorming, nominal group process, role playing, force field analysis, activity adaptation and informal socialization. We suggest that these strategies be used in conjunction with a system approach to activity processing.

Brainstorming to Generate Activity Options

During groups, the leader may be viewed by the patients as the expert and thus they expect you, the therapist, to assume total responsibility for determining what will happen during the group and the discussion that follows the activity experience. When it fits with the group maturity level it may be preferable to have group participants contribute their ideas to the group and be involved in group planning. The participants' contributions help to generate ideas, increase patient investment, and promote a feeling of group ownership. The sense is that this is "my group" and "I contributed to my group."

To promote the generation of ideas from group members, the leader may use structured techniques such as brainstorming, mind maping and imagining.

During *brainstorming*, a specific time period (five to ten minutes) is set aside for participants to spontaneously share thoughts, ideas and alternatives related to an identified topic and recorded on a flipchart or blackboard. The purpose is to generate as much information as possible during a brief time period. This information is then used by the group to select a focus activity or develop a discussion. For example, during an activity group for role clarification, the topic for the brainstorming period could be "roles in life." Group members would then, one at a time, spontaneously share ideas, feelings, values, etc., that relate to their roles; e.g. "I'm a father," "I'm frustrated, I have too many roles," "I am a friend, but want to be a lover," "My roles are determined by others," etc. The leader could then suggest that each group member make a personal-role collage using the themes suggested during brainstorming. The role-collage work period is then followed by a discussion about roles and how members feel about the way they fulfill their role responsibilities.

Once ideas are generated from brainstorming, the leader can help group members organize their spontaneous viewpoints. For instance, in the previous example, the participants' responses could be organized into categories such as "*Types* of roles we have in life-mother, father, friend, lover, worker, etc." or *Feelings* that our roles can cause — frustration, confusion, fulfillment, loss of control, etc."

After the categories have been identified, the leader helps the group choose the activity focus that best meets their needs and helps them share thoughts, feelings, and ideas that relate to the theme selected.

The brainstorming process may be outlined as follows:

1. Briefly describe the brainstorming process to the group.

2. Describe the discussion norms that apply; e.g., one person speaks at a time; any idea is acceptable, provided it doesn't hurt anyone else in the group.

    The goal is to generate a quantity of ideas not quality ideas, nothing is absurd; try not to be critical; ideas may be creative, practical, beyond the obvious, novel, etc.

3. Write the topic on the flipchart and give the group about five minutes to give input. The leader may assume responsibility for note-taking or can ask for a volunteer to record ideas on the flipchart.

It is preferable to write topics as positive statements. For example, instead of writing, "What is wrong with your job, life, personal appearance?" The leader could write "What would you like to change in your job, life, personal appearance?" Positive comments and the avoidance of value statements minimize defensive judgmental reactions, and promote a positive attitude toward problem solving (Carlisle and Murphy 1986, 42).

4. The recorder jots down the ideas during a 10-minute period.

5. Organize the ideas for discussion. See figure 9.1, for sample written structure, for organizing ideas. If you choose a specific written format, prepare the form in advance. (Carlisle & Murphy, 1986).

Matrix Ranking and Nominal Group Process to Prioritize Activities

During group tasks, (particularly those that involve problem solving) and group discussions, the leader may need to help the group set priorities in order to manage multiple group member needs or activity interests. Sometimes the therapist may choose the order of priorities and, when time and patient abilities permit, may ask the group to do so. Matrix ranking and nominal group process are two methods for setting priorities in a group.

Matrix ranking is more frequently used when the group size is small and there are a limited number of tasks. The intended outcome of ranking is group consensus (all members must agree rather than majority rule) on the priority. Since consensus is the goal, this method is not recommended for large groups.

The matrix ranking process has five steps:

1. Group members identify the tasks, activities or problems that they wish to work on during the group. The brainstorming process previously described may be used.

2. The group members' items generated in step one are listed on a flip chart, blackboard or graph paper.

3. Each item is compared with the other items and ranked. For example, for the items gardening, visiting museums, swimming, the order of preference might be: (1) swimming, (2) gardening, (3) visiting museums.

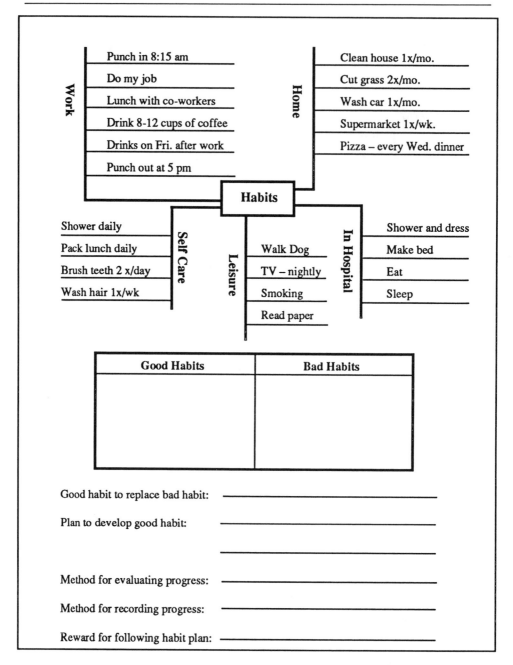

Figure 9.1   Mind Mapping Example

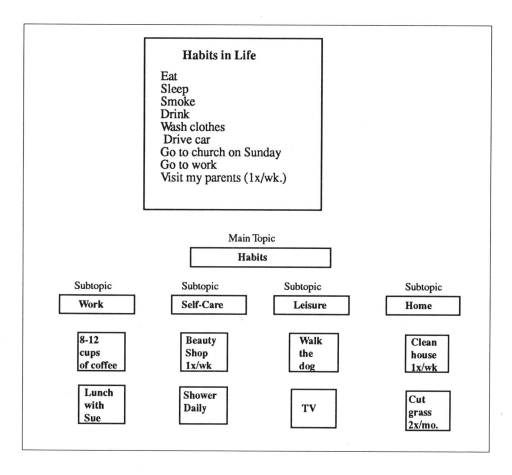

Figure 9.2 Brainstorming Example

4. The number of times each item is rated first, second, third, and so on, is counted and put in a matrix column, as in figure 9.3. Then place the total of each row in a total column. By comparing the numbers in the total column, the order of priority can be determined.

The *nominal group method* can be used with any size group and any number of items to be prioritized. Group member concensus is not required to determine task or discussion priorities. The nominal group method is a five-step process which requires all members to identify, rank, and prioritize the tasks or discussion topics they wish to pursue during the group.

The five step process includes:

Activity	First choice	Second choice	Third choice	Total Times Chosen
Bowling	1	4	5	10
Minature Golf	4	5	4	13
Movie	7	3	1	11
Swimming	1	1	3	5

The matrix indicates that the activity priority choice is: (1) minature golf, (2) movie, (3) bowling, and (4) swimming.

Figure 9.3   Matrix Ranking

1. Have each group member write the items he or she wishes to address on a three-by-five index card. This may be done before the group meets.

2. Ask each group member to identify his or her interests or concerns to the rest of the group. This can be done through a round-robin method (the group leader systematically goes around the circle and asks each member to contribute an item) or through brainstorming.

3. The leader then helps the group eliminate duplicate items, combine similar ideas, and review the finalized agenda list.

4. Have each group member select three items of importance from the final list. Once the three items are selected ask each member to rate each of the three items awarding 3 points to the most important, 2 points to the next most important, and 1 point to the least important. The ranking process is simplified if the participants use three-by-five index cards and hand them to the group leader.

5. The group leader then tallies the points awarded to each item. Tasks and topics with the highest number of points receive the highest priority. See Figure 9.4 for an example of nominal ranking.

Activity	1st choice	2nd choice	3rd choice	Total Points
Bowling	6 (18)	3 (6)	2 (2)	26
Minature Golf	4 (12)	4 (8)	1 (1)	21
Movie	4 (12)	4 (8)	4 (4)	24
Swimming	3 (9)	6 (12)	1 (1)	22

Note: The number of times chosen is weighted by multipling specific number of points for each choice; first choice earns 3 points, second earns 2 points and third earns 1 point. This nominal ranking example indicates that the activity priority is (1) bowling, (2) movie, (3) swimming and (4) minature golf.

Figure 9.4 Nominal Group Ranking

Generating Choices in Lower Maturity Groups

In groups where patients are limited in their ability to choose the activities they'd like to be involved in (or when the leader feels that options must be limited for other reasons), there can still be an element of choice in the selection of a group activity. As always, the message to convey is that you respect the participants, believe in their potential health, and accept the limitations they may have. One strategy is for the leader to allow limited choice. For example, "Would you prefer to work on our synchronized rhythms today, or pick from someone's favorite tapes and just listen, and share afterwards?" A variation on this is to introduce choices within the activity that the leader has selected. For example, "Today we'll spend our time finishing up the mural for Family Day. I'd like you to decide as a group if you'd like to take our supplies outside and work on the patio, or stay here in the clinic. We'll take a vote and let the majority rule."

Sometimes individuals who seem unable to make decisions or offer suggestions just need more time to organize their thoughts than what they are usually given. These participants may be able to respond if they are told ahead of time what kinds of choices they might be asked to make. For instance, the therapist may tell them before a group meeting (either at the previous group meeting, or closer to the time of the group session): "At our next meeting we'll be deciding where to have our spring picnic. Think about the places you've picnicked before and see if you have any places you'd like to suggest."

Cueing for Success

In the example just given, the therapist gives cues to help persons who have difficulty generating ideas. There are many ways leaders do this, often without realizing it. *Cueing* occurs when the therapist draws the patients' attention to the activity's attribute that needs to be focused on. Patients having problems organizing their involvement in activity can be assisted with such prompts as "Pay special attention to your breathing" or "As you critique this resume, try to see if you can tell that Jim has been a reliable worker."

The therapist can assist patients who have difficulty generating or expressing ideas by listening carefully and encouraging any movement toward appropriate expression. This is similar to cueing . For example, the patients are asked where they'd like to go on the public bus, and one hesitant member says softly, "I . . . I like to swim. . . . " The therapist helps this become an appropriate response when he or she jumps in and says "Good, getting exercise is important. What are some of the facilities for swimming that we can reach by bus. (pause) The YMCA? (another patient's response) Any others?"

Role Playing for Skill Practice

Therapeutic activity groups are a place where patients can learn and practice skills. One of the more frequent methods used for skill practice is role playing. The group environment provides a structured, safe environment for experimenting with new behaviors or learning to change old patterns. During group role playing, participants can learn from trial and error, experiment with varied behaviors, and practice for "real life situations"

The following guidelines may be used when planning a role-playing experience for activity groups.

1. Describe the role-playing experience. Include the specific behaviors that are to be learned and the performance criteria that are to be mastered. State the objectives of the role play, the reasons for the role-playing experience, and how the mastered behaviors can be applied to daily life.

   An introduction to a role-playing activity may sound like this: "Today, during the activity group, we will practice job interviews. Last time we met, you wrote your resume. Its now time to practice selling yourself to a potential employer. Please choose a partner that you want to work with and go sit together." The therapist then pauses, allows members to choose partners, and continues with the instructions and skill-practice periods.

2. Give specific role-playing instructions which identify the role and responsibility of each group member: "Next, you and your partner decide which of you will be the employer and which the applicant. [Pause] Now, during the next ten minutes, the 'applicant' is to stand and enter the employers' office, introduce him/herself, state the position that he/she is interested in, and pause for the 'employer' to ask questions. 'Employers' are to ask the 'applicant' to summarize his/her employment history."

3. Demonstrate the behaviors to be learned or the skills to be practiced. Demonstrations may be provided by the therapist (as role model) or by a brief film, video recording, or printed dialogue handout. In this example, the therapist could show a film of an employment interview, or ask a patient volunteer or co-therapist to do a role play in which employment interview skills are demonstrated.

4. Delegate role-playing responsibilities to each group member. If the group is relatively large, the leader may subdivide the group and have small groups plan several role plays. If there will only be one role-playing group that uses two or three group members, the other group members are observers.

   Observers should be given specific criteria to watch for during the role play and should be told that they will be expected to provide feedback to the group regarding the behaviors demonstrated or skills practiced. Avoid having too many observers, or give non role-playing members a specific observation assignment. In general, it is best to have active participants and provide skill practice. This often builds group members' confidence and can increase their satisfaction with the group experience.

5. Once the role play ensues, the group leader can coach players, but should not interfere with the flow of action. The leader may choose to observe the various role plays and make observation notes that can be shared with the entire group during the discussion that follows. When sharing observations, the leader may acknowledge good role models, contrast behavior approaches and skills, or bring up situations for group problem-solving. For example, when observing a role play the leader may pose questions: "Is it okay to ask about employment benefits during a job interview?" or "How much detail do you give about your personal life?"

6. When the role play is completed, the group leader facilitates a discussion in which group members share their observations and give feedback to the role players. The leader monitors the discussion to promote constructive criticism and prevent comments which are destructive to patient confidence or growth; (e.g. "that was stupid, that was terrible") If possible, when constructive criticism is given, act out the alternatives in a role play.

Force Field Analysis for Problem Solving

One method of problem solving in activity groups is force field analysis. (See Endnote #12) *Force field analysis* is a method for analyzing functional problems and identifying the forces which support or resist change. The analysis has six steps:

1. The leader identifies the behavior, dilemma, or performance that needs to be changed and writes it at the top of a blackboard. This can be thought of as defining the situation.

2. The leader writes the desired change (goal) at the bottom of the flip chart or blackboard.

3. The leader then facilitates a group discussion to identify the actions that support change and those that are barriers to change. Each support or barrier is listed on the flip chart: supporters on the right side and barriers on the left side.

4. The written format may also include a section of unclassified forces, that is, those factors which influence change but are not identified as supports nor barriers.

5. The group then rank-orders each of the forces that have been identified by the group. Before determining rank, the leader suggests that group members consider if the support forces can be easily implemented, if they can produce the desired change (quickly and with little effort and the most impact), and if they are capable of producing a long-lasting effect.

6. The group chooses the actions which will facilitate the desired change and accomplish the goal. Please see figures 9.5a and b for an example of the force field analysis.

Adapting Activities

Sometimes therapist-leaders find themselves in an activity group that doesn't seem to be going anywhere despite careful planning. Patients may

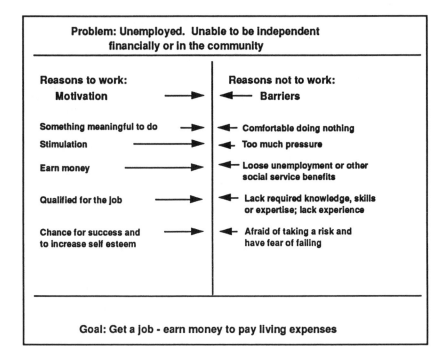

Figure 9.5a   Force Field Analysis. Content adapted from prevocational module. In Kramer (1984) SCORE: Solving Community Obstacles and Restoring Employment, New York, Haworth Press.

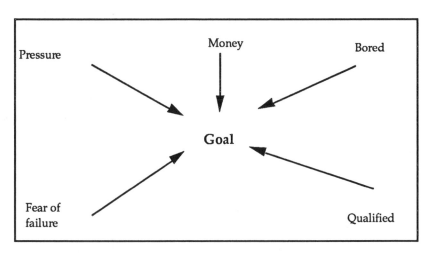

Figure 9.5b   Alternative representation of force field analysis.

be unresponsive, and it seems like "pulling teeth" to maintain interaction. Other times, participants may be trying to be involved, but have problems "catching on" to the activity. Often when there is a need for a change in the activity system, the therapist experiences it as a "tug" pulling in a direction different than the one he or she had been trying to take the group. One way to conceptualize this tug for activity adaptation is to see it as a healthy response to feedback within the system. We can remind ourselves that a functioning open system is responsive, and it changes as it needs.

Not everyone is equally adept at making on-the-spot changes in an activity during the group session. This is true for the patients as well as the group leader. On occasion, either may resist a change in plans. However, some of the most meaningful activity experiences have resulted when the therapist was able to discern and respond to the need to modify an activity and/or the approach to the activity.

Adapting activities can involve an endless number of strategies. Therapists who are skilled at adapting activities ask themselves the kind of questions that follow, though they may not have their questions posed as concretely as they are presented here.

1. *Is the activity, (as presented) too complex?* Could it be broken down into more manageable steps? Is the degree of complexity and the attention to detail too demanding? Is too much remembering involved?

2. *Is the activity too simple?* Sometimes patients lose interest when they are ready to handle more of a challenge than they are being given. Although activities can be made more complex, therapists usually try to avoid adding superfluous detail or creating unnecessary obstacles just for the sake of complexity. Oftentimes an activity that under normal circumstances is too simple needs to be replaced by a different task.

3. *Is the activity overstimulating or overwhelming?* Withdrawal is one way patients manage activity overload. Some patients may become scattered or behave inappropriately. Stimulation comes in many forms; including the general commotion of persons moving about; laughter, visual, tactile, auditory or other excessive input; novelty; being asked to manage multiple ideas or questions, and feelings or thoughts that are anxiety-producing.

4. *Would a change of pace be useful?* Changing the rhythm in a group (e.g. asking a highly active group to be quiet and contemplative; or mobilizing a group that has been sedentary) helps create a new focus, and can help to recharge energy. Time-outs, snack breaks and short walks can all help.

At times, therapists become predictable in the way they speak and present an activity. One option is to let someone else in the group introduce or guide the activity process. Later, the group might want to talk about how the group experience seemed different with this change.

5. *Would emphasizing a different sensory system be useful?* If a group seems to be non-responsive to material given in a handout, the therapist might tell them to put the handouts away and ask for verbal sharing. In the opposite situation, patients who are having difficulty responding verbally might be asked to jot their thoughts down on paper. Dimming the lights can enhance the auditory sense; shutting eyes can enhance both auditory and tactile input, and so on.

6. *Is the group having trouble attending to this activity because of some unfinished business?* On occasion several group participants may have concerns left over from other ward events, from home, or from events of the previous group meeting. If the therapist is aware of the unfinished issue, he or she might choose to give the membership a chance to respond and work though it. For instance, the therapist might say, "I can see you're having trouble getting into the poetry I brought. I'm wondering if some of you are worried about Mr. Jones [a group member]. I can tell you that he did have a heart attack, but is in stable condition." After giving the group a chance to voice their concerns, the therapist suggests, "Rather than work with the material I brought, perhaps you'd like to get out some construction paper and we can make a card to give him. The 'poets' in the group might want to add their own verses."

   Not every issue, can be handled like this in an activity group, but keeping abreast of ward and personal issues and facilitating closure when possible, enhances the therapist's ability to use the group time in a way meaningful to the participants.

7. *Has the activity gone on too long?* An activity that leaders believe will hold the group's interests for twenty or thirty minutes may fail to do so in actual practice. Having a repertoire of activities or exercises to draw from can be a life saver. Another option is to let the group know that you have misjudged the amount of time needed, and ask the members how they would like to use the time remaining.

8. *Does the activity need more time to be developed?* It is often only with experience that therapists learn that certain activities really need

more time than what has been allowed. Remembering that — for the next time the activity is used, may be the best you can do. Or, with some activities, you might ask the group to stop for this session, and assure them, that the activity will be brought to completion at the next meeting.

9. *Why do we have to do* this *activity?* Therapists pick particular activities in part because they provide the group with a chance to learn or practice particular skills or to gain specific information. But if the therapist has misjudged the participants interests at a given time, the group may be unenthusiastic about what is being proposed. If, for instance, the group members need an activity that involves heavy work patterns but they groan at the thought of digging a garden, maybe a spontaneous tug-of-war could be substituted.

10. *Am I taking too much (or too little) responsibility?* Given that we all do our conscientious best to support a positive group, we at times get so caught up in trying to improve the activity, that we discover we're doing all the work. In some cases it is very appropriate to throw the responsibility back to group members and ask them to initiate changes if they are unhappy with the group's focus or progress. In other instances, therapists may have assumed the group to be more mature than it is, and the therapist may need to intervene to facilitate the group's process.

Informal Socialization to Support Friendships

Some groups begin or end with an informal socialization period, which encourages participants to relate to each other in a nonstructured situation and develop friendships. The informal setting may include background music and serving refreshments, which should be served preferably when they will not interfere with the activity or discussion. Serving them before the activity creates a socializing period that can be the group's warm up. Serving them after the activity gives the participants time to wind down from the activity experience. They may feel more comfortable socializing informally after a structured activity, and can benefit from seeing the therapist-leader relax and relate casually. Sometimes, refreshments that meet the group members' needs or customs are served, as in a coffee break or afternoon tea, or when cookies and milk are provided and evoke memories of home.

General Guidelines for Discussion

As the focus activity comes to a conclusion, many groups will begin a discussion wrap-up. During this wrap-up, the leader uses group discussion and activity processing to help the group gain an understanding of the outcome of the group activity and reinforce the knowledge and skills they have gained from it.

Planning the Discussion

As part of the activity group protocol, the leader can consider the ideal conditions and the strategies to use during the discussion when processing the activity. The group discussion needs a recognized leader; therefore, if you have a co-leader, specify which one of you has primary responsibility for introducing the discussion and processing the activity. When planning for discussion, it is advisable to allow more time than what you think is necessary to allow all participants who wish to participate. It is useful to have identified priorities for discussion, to focus on the issues of importance. Otherwise, time can run out, and the activity group does not reach closure.

The therapist should also consider how the surroundings can be expected to influence discussion during the group experience. As with other aspects of the group session, the environment needs to provide physical and psychological comfort and have minimal distractions. Consider heat, ventilation, placement of furniture, and resources available to structure the discussion (blackboard, newprint, etc.). A comfortable environment with chairs arranged in a circle, in small groupings, or around a table will support patient interaction.

The leader may also wish to develop a few discussion questions that relate to the group activity. These are used to stimulate dialogue as well as reinforce the goals of the activity experience.

Opening the Discussion

After the activity, when the discussion portion of the group begins, the leader identifies the boundaries for interaction: "We have fifteen minutes left during which we can share our views of today's activity experience." The leader may also reiterate norms for confidentiality, respect for everyone's opinions, etc. in order to reinforce the climate of trust, acceptance, and support. Specific ground rules may be established. For instance, participants may be asked to avoid critical comments, and may be encouraged to look at issues from multiple perspectives. Patients may be asked to make

"I" statements rather than "you" statements. For example, "*I* had problems working with you on the mural when you kept the paint bucket by your side" rather than "*You* are selfish," or "you don't share." Or, the group may be asked to focus their comments specifically on events that occurred within the group activity session, as opposed to events at home or elsewhere. The leader maintains a safe, nonjudgmental, informal atmosphere in which all members are encouraged to interact.

Facilitating the Discussion

Throughout the discussion the leader tries to draw out and support participants, monitors talkative members to prevent monopolization, recognizes varying opinions in an unbiased manner, and helps the group sort through differing opinions and stay on track. As an important adjunct to this process, the leader is aware of his or her responsibility to help patients to manage their fear or anxiety. When individuals confront or disagree with each other, the leader needs to assess whether they can cope with it and whether the discussion, at this point, is of benefit to the entire group. The leader does not want any patient to leave the group filled with remorse over what he or she has said or done. Nor does the leader allow destructive feedback. It is helpful if the leader notices signals that suggest that the discussion or feedback process is getting out of control for anyone, so that he or she can intervene via a protective or boundarying response.

The discussion leader's primary guide: remember, in leader-participant interactions, the patient is central. Therefore, leader responses are based upon what is best for the patient and the whole group, and what needs to be achieved in the therapeutic activity.

The group leader can facilitate the activity discussion and help the members organize information by giving periodic summaries during the discussion and by using guided questions discussed earlier. The leader should check with group members to be certain they have closure on an issue, and then guide the discussion to the next topic. An important boundarying device is the leader's bringing the discussion back to its focus when members throw in distracting agenda items.

The leader can also help the group organize nonverbal information. For example, the leader can verbalize affirmation for the patient who nods in approval or help a member who is looking downward and saying nothing by putting his or her feelings of disapproval, rejection or fear into words.

If group members tend to be shy or silent, the group leader may be more active initially during the first half of the group or first few sessions of a series. The leader can present topics for discussion, give examples that relate to the activity experience, and identify the problems that participants are trying to resolve.

In addition to being accepting of the various levels of participation, the leader must remember that much can be learned through listening and that although some members remain silent, they may still be benefiting from the activity and discussion experience.

Closing the Discussion

When bringing the discussion to a close, the group leader may summarize the views stated and contrast points of agreement and disagreement. The leader may have the participants evaluate the activity group experience; the leader may help the group consider future plans.

For example, when closing a relaxation and leisure skills group, the therapist might ask the participants to describe the difference between active and passive relaxation. Then he or she might ask the participants to talk about some of the leisure interests they identified on their interest check list. The therapist then might suggest that the agenda for the next group be, "Budgeting for pleasure" and ask the participants to come to the next meeting with a list of leisure activities they want to pursue while in the hospital and in the community after discharge.

When using these discussion guides, the leader also incorporates specific strategies for processing an activity. These are discussed next.

Systematic Activity Processing

Activity processing is a guided discussion in which the therapist tries to help patients recognize how the activity relates to circumstances in their own lives. Not every activity group will end with an activity processing discussion; however it is an aspect of group discussion specific to activity groups.

Although the purpose of an activity may be apparent to us, some patients can not understand the relationship between an activity experience and what they hope to achieve through treatment. Therefore, it may be important to plan for a specific time for processing. The extent of activity processing can also be influenced by the depth of interaction and understanding the therapist hopes the participants to achieve, as well as the time available. The therapist may choose to summarize the relationship between the goals of the group and the activity, or may facilitate a discussion about the activity, with the intention of helping patients achieve insight into their behavior in the group.

When processing an activity during a group discussion, the therapist uses his or her observations of the group response as a whole as well as those of the individuals in the activity group. These observations can be processed systematically. The therapist can relate observations to the elements of the previous systems decribed in this text: the person system (e.g. personality, motivation, symptoms, strengths, problems, autonomy, social roles, etc.); the environmental/cultural system (e.g. group, hospital, community, cultural values, rules, etc.); and the activity system (e.g. cognitive, social, creative, structured, educational, simulated, playful, etc.) One or more of these systems may be the focus of the discussion. The therapist may also emphasize specific elements of the system in order to achieve a therapeutic goal.

In general, the therapist facilitates a discussion in which the purpose of the activity and the "here and now" activity events are related to the intended group outcome.

For example: The therapist has allowed 45 minutes for each participant to create a collage; the theme is reminiscence; the goal is to review one's life history and share some of life's significant events with other members of the group. The therapist opens the discussion: "During the activity time I noticed that participants worked sporadically, perferring to visit with each other and reminisce privately. Although you have done so privately, I want you now to share some of the significant events in your life with other group members. Who wants to begin?" (Pause) After individual members have shared significant events, the leader identifies those that seem most significant to the group.

After hearing the participants' responses, the therapist can ask the group to make a list of the most frequently cited events and suggest that these events have importance to the group.

> "Your responses show that most of you feel good about
> your work contributions throughout life, but miss your work and
> family life of the past. It looks as though you are trying to decide
> how to establish new networks of friends and workers."

If the group hour is over, the therapist might suggest a topic for the next group meeting (e.g., "establishing networks" or "how to bring 'healthy stress' into one's life") or the therapist might relate the themes to one of the other systems that influence the group outcome. For example,

(a) Relate the responses to the milieu or the environment (here, the hospital environment); e.g., "You have commented on the lack of stimulation you feel when you're at home. How do you feel about the level of activity here in the hospital?"

(b) Relate the themes to the group goals and the person system; e.g., "Today you have had an opportunity to reminisce and share some of your life history with group members. Reviewing your experiences is the first step in identifing your accomplishments and strengths. Next I'd like each member of the group to share one of their personal strengths."

(c) Relate the activity experience and discussion to the individual's goals and how the activity supports their achievement; e.g. "Now that we have all shared some of the significant events in our life, I'd like you to talk with the person on your right, beginning with ____ [state a name]. Share with your partner what you did in the group today that relates to your personal goal you hope to achieve while in the hospital [day care program]." Patients may say that they were able to speak in front of a group, that the group activity helped them relax and so on.

(d) Establish a link between the activity and the community environment to which the patient will return; e.g, "In the group today, we have shared our histories, identified a personal strength, and suggested topics for future groups. How do the outcomes of today's group relate to your life in the community?" If the patients cannot make this connection between treatment and community life, the therapist may provide prompts:

"How might you use your personal strengths when you return home (to work)?" "When we first meet someone, we usually share some of our personal history. From your experience today, what would you like to share with a potential friend?"

These relationships are drawn to increase the participants' self awareness, and to provide an opportunity for patients to share and learn from each other.

After the activity has been processed and its relationship to specific individual or group goals discussed , the therapist closes the group. He or she may state, "The group is over for today. Thank you for your participation," and state when the next group meets, "I'll see you tomorrow at 10:00 a.m." Or he or she may ask the participants to make a personal committment to change.

Group Closure Through Personal Commitment

Some groups end with each patient making a personal commitment to change specific behaviors or practice new skills before the next meeting. A personal commitment is like a therapeutic contract made between a therapist and a patient. Although the personal commitment may be made verbally, it is often better to have each member make it in writing.

Written personal commitments are positive statements which identify specific behaviors worked on in the group. Statements are written in the present tense and can often be memorized by the patient. The group may jointly write commitment statements; these are then recorded on a blackboard or a flip chart. Each group member then writes it on a three-by-five card and takes it with them to repeat the commitment twice a day. The card may also be used to record the times the patient meets his or her commitment.

Leaders usually help participants state the commitment in positive behavioral terms. The commitment describes a specific goal that addresses a patient problem or general discomfort. For example, when a patient states, "I avoid people and don't like to look them in the eye. . . . I have never been able to look at people. I wish I could," a positive format would be:

Personal Committment: I will make eye contact with persons that I see on the nursing unit and say 'hello'. If I see a new patient, I'll introduce myself and shake hands with the new acquaintance. I will record the times I say "hello" on the back of this card.

Chapter Summary

To promote the patient's participation, learning, and understanding of the value of the activity, the group leader plans the activity structure and method of processing before the group experience. However, this plan may need to be modified as the group ensues to accomodate the unpredictable and unique interactions that occur among the group elements (therapist, participant, activity and environment).

Summary of Group Throughput

Once the elements of the group come together and the group ensues, the therapist structures the experience as needed to keep the group active, organized, and boundaried, and monitors the process that develops. The group, activity structure, and process together create the throughput of the system. As stated previously, the throughput can be understood as the "how and why" of the group. How are the input elements influencing one another? Why is this process occurring or what influences the process of interaction during the group?

When monitoring the throughput of the group, the leader views and seeks to understand the "whole" created by the activity group experience within the context of the greater environment. Understanding the "whole" picture helps the leader adapt the activity as needed to achieve goals and to facilitate discussion and feedback during the group experience.

While monitoring the activity experience to get a sense of the "whole" group and its process the leader can ask:

1. *Are the goals expressed by the group members compatible with those of the group plan?*

   When patients are appropriately referred to and selected for the group, they can more easily relate to the group experience and see the group as a means to achieve personal goals. When goals are not compatible it may feel as if there is a "tug of war" going on in the group as the leader tries to facilitate participation but the members are not interested in or seem resistant to the activity. Additionally, the therapist may ask *Do patients understand the relationship between the group experience and their overall treatment plan?* Even when patients are actively involved in the experience, they may not understand the purpose, nor the benefit, of the activity group. One thing the leader can do is use processing to increase the patients' understanding of the benefits of activity.

2. *What is the feeling of the group?*

   Participants react to each as well as to the activity and the leadership. These reactions contribute to the formation of a group feeling. This "feeling" encompasses the emotional climate as well as communicates the expectations and acceptance of participants for themselves and each other. For example, the overall tone in a group may be experienced as competitive, relaxed, or lethargic. Another vital contributor to the group climate is the feeling of "groupness" or the 'esprit de corps' as members experience themselves as belonging to a larger whole.

3. What *is the purpose or function of the activity in this group?*

The activity is used to facilitate interaction, promote learning, and enable the achievement of individual and group goals. If the activity is serving these purposes, the leader implements the activity experience as planned. If not, the leader considers ways of adapting the activity. He or she may do this independently or in collaboration with the group participants.

4. *How are the methods of communication meeting individuals' and the group's needs?*

The leader evaluates the content of verbal and nonverbal interactions as well as the communication style of the participants. The relative success of communication within the group helps to determine the adequacy of group interaction and influences the feedback of the group system. If group communication and feedback is minimal or substandard, the leader tries to identify what prevents group interaction, and responds accordingly.

5. *What roles are participants assuming?*

During the group, members can assume varied task and maintenance group roles. These roles influence the individual participant's learning as well as the integrity and effectiveness of the activity group. Roles can be formally assigned or informally assumed as the membership spontaneously interacts during the activity experience. These roles and how they are fulfilled also contribute to the social network influencing the group outcome.

6. *How does the leader style influence the group and activity process?*

As described previously, situational leadership allows the group leader to respond to the maturity level of group members and adapt to the changes, interactions, and needs expressed during an activity group experience. The situational style depends on feedback from the membership and treatment environment, as well as the leader's expertise.

7. *How do participants view my leadership?*
   Patients may have a different view of the role or effectiveness of the leader. Patients may expect the leader to take control or may resist his or her guidance. They may appreciate or avoid the opportunity for shared authority. Because of the varied expectations, these views may need to be discussed in order for the group to operate more effectively and move on to achieve goals.

8. *Do participants understand what is expected of them?*
   Activities may evoke many responses from the group participants: e.g., comfort with the activity or tension at the throught of trying something unfamiliar; there may be pleasure at the opportunity to be creative, play, and socialize, or dislike for the social nature of the group activity. Because of the variety of responses that an activity can engender, the leader may need to discuss the expectations for participation. For example, when group members are not involved in the activity, the leader may feel that they are resistant or minimally committed to treatment. However, before making this assumption, the leader can try to determine if the participant understands the group's expectations for him or her.

9. *How do participants seem to view each other?*
   The picture we hold of ourselves may be similar to or different from the image we project to others. The extent to which the personal and public self agree often influences the group and activity process. During activity groups when participants verbalize their views, learning is enhanced since there exists an opportunity to resolve incongruities.

10. *Do the activity and discussion processes within the group complement each other?*
    As described earlier in this text, we can think of a group continuum in which the emphasis upon activity or discussion will help to identify a group as a verbal, task or, therapeutic activity group. In therapeutic activity groups priority is given to activity, as well as to discussion. Both activity and discussion are valued because they support and reinforce one another to promote the group outcome.

We next turn our attention to this third part of the activity group system model, that of group outcome.

10
Group Outcome: A Blending of Task and Group Maintenance Functions, Feedback, and Termination

Focus Questions:

1. What outcomes occur as a result of the therapeutic activity group experience?
2. How is the effectiveness of the group outcome determined?
3. How does the dynamic process of the group system influence the group outcome?
4. Which systems of documentation and communication can be used to record and communicate the group outcome?
5. How does feedback influence the group and treatment systems?
6. What occurs when the group terminates?

Group Outcome

The group outcome was described as more than the sum of the group's parts by Lewin (1951) and von Bertalanffy (1968). As discussed earlier, Lewin saw the outcome as the equilibrium resulting from opposite forces: some forces push to keep the status quo; others push for change. Bales (1950, 1955, 1958) described outcome as a balance between task and maintenance functions; Homans saw the outcome as an exchange between the rewards and costs of interpersonal interaction and, a direct proportion between group input and output (Homans, et.al, 1961).

All these system-based theories suggest that the group outcome moves to maintain an equilibrium between the elements of the group system and between the group system, and other systems in the environment (open-system equilibrium). However, von Bertalanffy did not feel that the equilibrium model applied to open systems. He believed that the equilibrium model was more consistent with the ideas of tension reduction and maintenance of the status quo rather than with the dynamic process of an open system. (von Bertalanffy 1968, 40)

Open or living systems are distinguished by the ability to change and become more complex. One can look at the group's outcome as the relationship between changes effecting the group and elements that remain unchanged. If too much in the group's elements and process were to change, there would be little to hold the group together as a system. Also, if many elements change, the participants may have too much to assimilate. The quest becomes one for demonstrable changes that represent the goals of the group and individual members, while maintaining adequate consistency within the system.

Change

The change that occurs within individuals or within the group may barely be noticeable, or may be easily seen. Change may occur in one or more elements of the group system and usually all elements are influenced by their being brought together for a common experience. In general, the change process is reflected in the person's or group's ability to manage themselves better, relate to others, and participate successfully in the environment.

Participant Changes

When individuals change they may see themselves differently, relate to others differently, may be more active in the environment, or may try new approches to problem solving and risk taking . Although the changes that result from the group experience can be dominant in any of the "subsystems" of personhood (psychological, physical, cognitive, spiritual or social) the reader is reminded that any one change inevitably affects the person as a whole, as well as the larger systems of which he or she is a part.

While participating in a therapeutic activity group, individuals may verbalize new thoughts or attitudes, or behave differently. Or they may demonstrate a new skill, acknowledge a feeling of group ownership, or show concern for another participant. When new attitudes and behavior are not evident during the group experience, they may emerge when the participants interact in other social systems. However, some changes are much more difficult to see, such as those related to subtle developments in reasoning, spirituality, understanding and emotion.

If you want to verify behavior change resulting from a program, you will need to do an initial performance evaluation before the group experience begins. Then use this information to establish a behavior baseline and determine behavioral objectives describing the performance goals desired. The patient then participates in groups that are compatible with the targeted behavioral objectives. When the group program is completed, the participant may be retested, or other methods may be used to determine if the desired outcomes were achieved. These outcomes are then documented.

Group Leader Changes

The group leader, as well as the participants, is influenced by the activity group experience. The leader may gain a heightened personal awareness and knowledge that will increase his or her clinical expertise. However, the leader's personal experiences are seldom the focus of the group. What the leader has learned about him or herself is shared during the group only when this disclosure can promote the group process and development, or is otherwise of benefit to patients.

Reader Activity

As difficult as defining changes is for patients who have sensed their occurrence, it is often just as difficult for the therapist who feels different as a result of the group experience. Occasionally, there is an "Aha!" experience, when an insight suddenly crystallizes, or a piece of information becomes evident. However, it is probably through one's participation in several social or clinical groups that the evolution (not revolution) of personal change can be identified.

If you have been involved in a group (social, clinical, classroom, or other) over the past three months or longer, give an example that would fit the following:

1. Something you know about yourself (e.g. belief, philosophy or bias) that was influenced by the group experience.

2. Something you believe about others that was gained during the group.

3. A behavior you have intentionally altered due to the feedback given to you during the group.

4. A personal behavior not intentionally altered but somehow seemingly different as a result of your group involvement.

5. An increase in clinical expertise, knowledge or skill that came as a
   result of the group.

Environmental Change

The environment in which the activity group occurs may undergo
changes during the group experience. For instance, the group atmosphere
may take on specific characteristics that can enhance or interfere with the
group's meeting their goals. The group can engender a supportive atmosphere that meets individual as well as group needs (gains in participant
self confidence and skill development, with concurrent increase in the
group's prestige in the treatment community). Conversely, the group may
promote an atmosphere which encourages individuals to blame one another and emphasize the faults of individuals or the treatment system.
Changes within the group environment usually spill over into the other
related environmental systems. This is often seen when a patient has
positive feelings about his or her involvment with a specific medical or
social service. Patients tend to carry these positive feelings into the other
medical or social services they contact. If a patient has a negative experience, he or she may disavow all medical and social service providers, and
the "system" as a whole.

The group may also have an effect on the treatment milieu where it
occurs. A tumultuous group is likely to be "felt" on the ward long after it
ends, and it is not unusual for treatment staff to follow up individuals after
such a group session. To follow up and work through some of the unresolved issues that may exist after an activity group, the staff needs a sense
of what occurred during the activity group.

Group follow-up is one important reason for documenting the group
experience. Documentation needs to be available to those who come into
the milieu and work with participants after the group has concluded. This
communication and follow up are part of the mechanism of feedback in
the treatment system.

Change in Activity

The activity may result in a specific end product, or may have acted
as a learning experience, promoting group process and individual change.
The activity planned may have been used differently or adapted by the the
group. As discussed, such flexibility enables the activity to proceed in a way
that better meets both of individual and group needs.

Resistance to Change

Although all group system elements are subject to change during the activity group, all elements may also be resistant to change. Resistance to the group experience is likely occurring when participants show little interest in the activity, refuse to participate, choose to be silent or passively involved, repeatedly request to leave the group early, or attend the group only at the insistence of the staff.

The treatment milieu and therapist-leader may also resist change. Think of an occasion where a group in which you were involved, made a recommendation to a boss, a teacher, or institution that something in the routine should be changed. You may or may not have felt the suggestion was well received, and wondered if change would result.

Resistance to change is influenced by the participant's need to maintain personal identity and avoid a threat to integrity. Take the following example of the group resisting feedback.

During an activity group that uses teams to help participants learn to manage competition, the losing team blames their loss on the leader's inability to give clear instructions. The team members won't accept the group feedback that indicates that they neither had a team plan nor did they cooperatively work together. They resist looking at their team behavior, want to avoid feeling inferior to the other team, and are using the leader as a scapegoat rather than considering another way to work together.

Resistance may be a sign that the participants are evaluating the way a proposed change affects them. Does the change meet their own needs? Is it compatible with their values and interests? How will it influence their ability to cope with daily life and their ability to adapt to the situations they confront? Some participants may need time to understand the activity experience and how it has affected them. They are not resisting further involvement as originally assumed, but are taking time to process the experience.

Leadership and the Change Process

Leaders, when considering their role in the change process, evaluate how much they helped the group maintain a sense of continuity and "groupness" while fostering an experience that allowed for desired treatment outcomes. As leaders manage this balance between continuity and change they may review their role in the change process by asking:

1. Did I provide an effective leadership style? A style that helped to establish and maintain boundaries while being open to desired change?

2. Did I sense when participants desired a change and did I help persons move toward goal accomplishment during the activity group?

3. Did I promote an atmosphere that encouraged risk taking? A safe environment with adequate stimuli and support to minimize the discomfort of risk, but challenging enough to promote learning?

4. Did I build a bridge from the activity experience to the goals of the group and those desired in everyday life?

5. Did I facilitate communication and participation in the activity?

6. Did I help the group use the activity as a resource for problem solving? When problem solving, did I help the group define the goal and identify the issues and possible solutions? Did I provide the group with boundaries by setting a time limit for responding to the situation? Did I help the group make a commitment to change?

7. Did I provide reinforcements for the risks taken during the activity group?

8. Did I encourage feedback among participants?

9. Once goals were achieved, did I help the group reach closure and disengage?

Answers to these and other leader questions can help identify the forces that help promote change and the forces that maintain stability and continuity. These forces are reflected in the outcome of the group, and they influence the feedback that supports the group's existence.

Outcome – Group Development and Maintenance

As the various elements of the group change, the group depends on influences that help maintain the group's structure and support its future existence. The group is maintained by both internal and external influences. The internal influences include the group norms, factors supporting cohesiveness, the evidence of therapeutic gains, and the level of group development. These also affect the accomplishment of tasks and the feedback that contributes to the external factors maintaining the group. External influences by which the group is maintained include its history and the recognition it receives in the treatment milieu.

The group history develops over time and usually has an oral tradition. That is, participants learn about the group and its values from things told to them by previous group members, as well as from treatment staff. This oral history attests to the viability of the group and tends to increase the attraction of new members to the group.

In addition to depending on the group's history, the leader can influence the group maintenance with an established structure. For instance, having frequent meetings, a specific meeting place, and an identified time in the treatment program schedule all tend to contribute to the group's continuity and stability. The benefits of group structure are readily apparent in such programs as Alcoholics Anonymous or Narcotics Anonymous, which meet in community settings.

The leader also helps maintain the group when he or she promotes participant "ownership" of the group. This is done by reflecting questions directed to the leader back to the membership and helping the participants identify their common interests, concerns, and needs. Participants tend to feel ownership when the leader role is shared with the membership. Shared leadership can increase member participation and cooperation, sharing of feelings, mutual support and satisfaction.

As the group evolves through the dual functions of facilitating maintenance and change, the leader, participants, and significant others begin to evaluate the overall treatment effectiveness of the activity group as a treatment tool.

Outcome — Group Effectiveness

There are multiple criteria that can be used to evaluate the outcome of the activity group and determine its effectiveness. The effectiveness of the group as a whole can be based upon opinions from those within or outside of the group. When a group is over, one is likely to hear comments such as, "That was a good group" "I'm glad that's over," "That was fun," or any number of personal reactions from the participants and leader. These reactions are usually related to the participants' standards, expectations, interests, values and needs, and how well the group experience has met these.

Participants' Evaluation

When the group is over, group members base much of their evaluation of group effectiveness upon their immediate feelings and sense of accomplishment. For instance they may notice that they feel relaxed, or were not too uncomfortable, that they didn't offend anyone, that there were no disagreements, that they had fun, learned something new and so on. Beyond these immediate reactions, participants may reflect on results of group effectiveness through a more formal mechanism.

Individual group members decide if the activity experience has helped them achieve the goals that they have established for the particular group session or the treatment program. The group leader can solicit the membership's opinion either through a request for feedback during the group summary ("What did you gain from the activity experience today?") or by using a more formal system in which the participants are asked to complete a questionnaire at the end of the group or series of groups. Possible questionnaire items include: "What was most/least helpful during the activity group?" or "What have you achieved/learned/changed as a result of the activity experience?" A check list of items such as those in Figure 10.1, may be used.

Leader's Evaluation

The leader will also make a judgment regarding the effectiveness of the group. Leaders may comment, "The patients worked together," "They responded well to the activity," "They were cooperative," "Group was fun today," "I learned . . . ," or any number of reactions. Beyond these immediate reactions, leaders tend to contrast one group experience with another to judge the group's effectiveness. Therapists have often said that even when they use the same group activity or plan, the group outcome varies. The leader evaluates whether the group outcome is similar to the one which was expected, given the group plan and previous experiences.

One way to validate the leader's perceptions or assumptions is to check them out with the group members. When bringing closure to the activity group the leader might state, "I appreciate the cooperation that I saw during the cooking group today and wonder if you are pleased with the way that the party preparations were made today? Please take a minute to share your view of what you accomplished today."

Another possibility is to discuss the group experience and its outcome with one's supervisor, co-leader, or other team members. This feedback can be supportive and confirm one's opinion, or it may help the leader see alternatives for facilitating a more effective response. This discussion can be particularly useful when the leader is feeling frustrated by the group's outcome.

Evaluation by Significant Others

The outcome of the group is also evaluated by the significant others in the participants' lives. Family members and staff members frequently base their assessment of the group on the participants' behavior outside. They often want participants to be more cooperative and adaptive, or are pleased when patients have a brighter affect or show new interests. Signifi-

---

Group Outcome Survey

Please answer each of the following questions.

1. The most helpful aspect of the group was:

    _____

2. The least helpful aspect of the group was:

    _____

3. During the group I felt:

    _____

4. During the group I learned:

    _____

5. Do you still use the knowledge and skills that you learned in the group? Please explain:

    _____

6. Did you feel free to participate in the activity? In the discussion?

    _____

7. How did others in the group help you?

    _____

8. In general, I felt that the group experience was: (circle one)

    very   poor   mediocre   good   very   excellent
    poor   good

    _____

9. Comments:

    _____

10. Suggestions:

    _____

Figure 10.1   Group Outcome Survey

cant others can provide feedback regarding changes in the patient's performance and indicate whether or not the behavior is similar to that learned in activity groups.

The opinions of others can be elicited verbally or through a written format. Questionnaires may be sent to family members. The questions are related to the goals of the group and typically ask significant others to describe or rate the participant's performance since the group experience. Sometimes such questions are a part of an overall program evaluation conducted at the conclusion of a patient's participation, or they may be part of a follow-up study six months to a year after treatment is discontinued.

Another avenue for evaluating the effectiveness of the group experience is to meet with the identified group consultant and discuss the group plan, process, and outcome, as described or recorded by the leader. Some settings have a treatment program review committee which can also serve as a source of feedback.

Some settings include a brief (10-15 minute) wrap up with staff members and other team members in which they process the group experience as well as identify strategies and plans for future therapeutic activity groups. The patient group may or may not be invited to listen to this staff critique.

Evaluation by the Treatment Team

On a personal level, treatment team members may view therapeutic activty groups as an element in the treatment system which gives them a brief reprieve from patient demands and time to catch up with paperwork and other related job responsibilities. The reader may have heard any number of comments such as "Thanks for taking the patients off the unit," I appreciated the time" or "Without interruptions, I finally got this done."

On the other hand, treatment team members are also sensitive when they are left with patients who have many unresolved issues and disruptive behavior that result in more work for them. These outcomes of the group experience also color the team members' view of group effectiveness.

The treatment team assesses the group outcome by the services provided in the treatment setting. They usually expect group outcomes to assist them in evaluation, treatment planning, and monitoring of progress. They expect leaders to give input into the master care plan and often ask for frequent feedback regarding patient performance.

In some settings, each treatment modality is asked to support research, quality assurance, and outcome studies. The methods of group documentation and feedback previously described in this chapter can contribute to these formal studies. In general, team members expect the activity group outcome to complement the other aspects of the treatment program and make their job easier.

Criteria for Group Effectiveness

Although each of the previously described group elements can be assessed according to very subjective criteria, there exist also objective criteria. Treatment professionals and specifically group leaders may be familiar with the criteria summarized in the literature.

Effective groups are those that have:

(1) identified goals which are understood by group members;

(2) accomplished the group task;

(3) have leadership that promotes participant responsibility and problem solving;

(4) have a broad based communication pattern that involves the majority of the group membership;

(5) an atmosphere of trust, support, safety, creativity and constructive controversy; and

(6) a pattern of growth and development that reflects group effectiveness, (Johnson & Johnson 1975, in Clark 1987, 12)

Ineffective groups do not meet the previous criteria, and more frequently emphasize conformity, have leadership that is controlling and strives to maintain the status quo. The members of an ineffective group may participate in the activity with little investment, show little interest in relating to one another, and tend to share ideas but often deny and/or ignore their feelings (Johnson & Johnson 1975 in Clark 1987, 12).

In summary, successful groups have members who arrive on time, attend the group consistently, and work cooperatively to achieve a goal. Participants may verbalize the value, importance, and benefit of the group, and they can disagree in a manner that promotes constructive feedback. This feedback stays within the group to promote individual change or maintain the group, and communicates the group outcome to the treatment system.

Feedback — Verbal and Written Communication of Group Process and Outcome

Feedback here refers to any information (verbal or written; audio tape or video recording) that (1) helps lead, guide, or direct the behavior of the group participants and the group as a whole, (2) helps maintain the group, and (3) goes out into the treatment system to communicate with significant others. (Sampson 1981, 123)

Feedback During the Group

During the group, feedback can bring unknown aspects of the participants' behavior to their attention and can inform them if their behavior matches their intentions. Feedback can facilitate learning and increase understanding when it is specific and descriptive. The guidelines for giving feedback are similar to those for any verbal exchange, as discussed in previous chapters.

The leader should encourage a timely feedback response that increases participant awareness and validates self-perceptions or encourages individuals to consider alternative viewpoints or solutions. Feedback should be descriptive in nature rather than evaluative: "I can't hear what you're saying," rather than "You don't speak loud enough." Or "I disagree with your viewpoint," rather than "You are wrong."

Descriptive feedback has a "here and now" focus and is direct and specific, not sarcastic or based upon broad generalizations. It is directed toward the behavior that the patient can change and is given in a caring, constructive manner. "In the group today, I noticed that you helped clean up the tables and put away supplies instead of waiting for other group members to do it for you," rather than, "I'm glad you did your share of the work for a change."

Once feedback is given the leader gives the patient a chance to respond and provides support for the exchange of responses. Participants are encouraged to continue relating in the here and now, and to avoid defensive or punitive reactions.

Verbal Report of Group Outcome

Verbal feedback is also given to other elements in the treatment system. Immediately following the therapeutic activity group, the therapist or co-therapists often will discuss the group outcome and highlight the group experience in a written or verbal summary to the other members of the treatment team who were not present. This communication with other treatment staff gives them the information they need for group follow up and promotes an integrated treatment approach.

The system for communicating group treatment events varies with the setting. Communication may occur at the change of shift or during an informal meeting. If the reader works in a setting that does not have an established communication system, the authors recommend that you establish a feedback system with the treatment team. The guides for written documentation which are outlined in this chapter may serve as a guide for the verbal summaries provided to treatment team members.

Written Documentation of Group Outcome

Those outcomes related to evaluation, treatment and research are usually recorded using a documentation system. The documentation may take the form of a narrative note, a problem oriented record system, or a specially structured form created for the individual treatment setting in which the group has occurred.

Narrative Group Note Format

In general the group narrative summary should include:

1. group descriptors: date, group title, group goals
2. description of the therapeutic activity
3. a list of patients in attendance
4. a brief summary of the group experience (process and outcome)

The summary of the group process may include:

a. the therapist observations of verbal and nonverbal communication and an interpretation and analysis of the group events; e.g., seating arrangment communication patterns, the participants' style of communication, and the memberships' response to leadership,
b. the task/activity and the problem solving that occurs during the group.

The summary of the group outcome describes the task accomplished, the level of group cohesion achieved and the level of closure achieved.

In addition to communicating with the treatment team about the outcome of the group as a whole, the leader also documents each participant's progress during the therapeutic activity. Progress may be recorded in a narrative note, on a check list, or on another structured format.

Date: November 10, 1989   **Group Title:** Managing change

Goals: To identify the recent and present changes that members have experienced; To identify the stable elements in their present situation, (familiar people, places, things and activities).

Activity: Mural Change and What it Feels Like

Patients in attendance: P. Smith, G. Lock, M. Davis, K. Dale J. Brook, L. Penny, C. Larson, P. Gregg

Summary: After a brief introduction to concepts of change, participants worked together cooperatively for **30** minutes to draw the change mural. After completing the mural, each participant shared recent changes he/she experienced and how change has affected his/her life. Everyone then completed the change work sheet in which they identified relationships, personal traditions, and habits that are stable and casn help them cope with change. These were shared with each other during a brainstorming session and summarized by the leader. In general, the group atmosphere changed from participants being scattered throughout the room to working with little interaction to interested in finding resources for coping with the changes they are experiencing.

Figure 10.2   Narrative Note Sample

A narrative notes describes the patient's response to the activity, leadership, other participants, and group experience in general. It may include a description of the role(s) the participant assumed in the group, peer response to the patient during the activity group, and a comparison to the patient's performance in previous groups. See figure 10.3 for an example.

P. D. (Patient's initials) participated in the 45-minute relaxation group to increase coping skills for pain management. After 15 minutes of progressive relaxation and a 15 minute guided imagery experience, she stated that she "felt less tense, still had pain but it was tolerable." She indicated that she would find it difficult to follow this routine at home due to the work demands there and the "noisy household." She was curt with another group member who would not accept her excuse of too much work. Establishing a relaxation routine at home will be discussed in future group sessions.

Figure 10.3   Sample Individual Note

The Structured Individual Progress Note

Given the shortage of staff, the need for efficient time management, and the use of technology, some treatment settings have developed structured formats which promote computerized documentation and the use of checklists or Likert scaling. These formats can decrease the time required for documentation and increase the time staff members are involved in patient treatment.

Kaplan has modified the structured progress note format used at a major medical center inpatient unit to identify the participant's perform-ance in directive groups (Kaplan1988). The form identifies the specific areas of function which are the treatment focus of the group, provides a scale for rating the level of performance, and includes a grid sheet for recording progress during a one-week period (Kaplan1988, 52, 53, 58). See figure 10.4 for an excerpt from the Kaplan progress note form.

A numerical system such as that used by Kaplan can facilitate the study of progress in outcome studies or research. A numerical format can be adapted to allow graphing of patient performance at the end of each week. This performance graph can give health care professionals a quick inter-pretation of the participant's progress.

Certificate of Completion

Groups which are based upon an educational frame of reference such as that described by Bachner (see the Community Cooking Group in part 2), document the group outcome by awarding a certificate of completion to each group participant. Participants who satisfactorily complete the group experiences or demonstrate a particular level of skill competency are given a certificate in recognition of their accomplishments. The cer-tificates resemble those which the reader may have received from continu-ing education courses.

Video Recordings

Video recordings may be used to document the group experience, then provide immediate feedback to the participants. Videos promote learning and provide audio-visual feedback to members on their partici-pation in the activity group. Group members are frequently surprised by the video portrayal of their physical appearance, style of interaction, and personal characteristics.

Prior to using audio or video recordings, the group leader needs the verbal and/or written permission of the group members. In most settings

Name:	Monday				Tuesday				Wednesday				Thursday			
Directive Group Progress Sheet Week of ———	Attend	Interact	Participate	Initiate	Attend	Interact	Participate	Initiate	Attend	Interact	Participate	Initiate	Attend	Interact	Participate	Initiate
(Patient's name)																

Reproduced with permission . Kaplan (1988)   New Jersey: SLACK Inc., 53.

Attention:
1   did not attend, highly distractable
2   attends 5 minutes or less
3   attends 5-15 minutes
4   attends 15-30 minutes
5   attentive entire 45 minutes

Participation:
1   uncooperative, resists involvement in activities
2   participates minimally
3   needs consistent support or structure to assure activity involvement; or is hyperactive
4   minimal assistance to cooperate actively in group activity
5   cooperates actively in all group activities without assistance

Initiation:
1   unable to volunteer activities on own
2   can choose between two alternatives
3   elaborates upon activity ideas with direct assistance
4   makes suggestions (but may be inappropriate)
5   suggests, explains, or demonstrates at least one group activity (spontaneous initiation)

Interaction:
1   did not respond verbally
2   minimal response or inappropriate response to direct question
3   moderate response to direct question or monopolizes
4   responds verbally to direct question and is appropriate
5   spontaneous and appropriate verbal responses to remarks or comments

Figure 10.4   Sample Structured Documentation.

patient consensus is required; those patients who refuse to give permission are allowed to leave the group. If the recordings are to be heard or viewed by persons other than those participating in the group, written permission from the group participants is required. The reader is encouraged to consult with the health setting's advisory board or patient advocate regarding the patient privacy act and release of responsibilities documents.

Outcome–Group Closure and Termination

Once the group task is accomplished the leader helps to bring closure to the group experience. *Closure,* the end of each group session, is the process that ties together what was learned and what was accomplished during the group. To achieve closure the leader helps the participants determine whether they met the group's goals, and if not, what prevented the group from accomplishing its task. Regardless of the level of group success, the leader seeks to end the group with an optimistic feeling that supports the participants' self- esteem and communicates that they are capable of success or mastery. Also, the leader may help the group understand what went wrong, and what they could do in the future to be more successful.

For some groups, task completion may also mean that it's time for the group to disband or terminate. Termination refers more to the ongoing group that finally ends after a series of sessions. However, in open groups where the membership changes constantly, formal termination may be ill-defined. Participants may leave the group because of discharge or because they or the leader determined that the group was not a useful treatment tool for them. In either case the group participants must say goodbye and cope with the process of separation. To separate, group members need time during the group to talk about their experience and what they have shared and learned. At termination, participants may also describe the fellowship they experienced and how they feel about their contributions to the group goals.

The ending of a group can cause multiple feelings: joy, accomplishment, sadness, relief, rejection, anger. All of these are feelings associated with those experienced with other endings in one's life. Therefore during termination, the leader will help the participants share their reactions to separation, review their accomplishments, and focus on how the ending of this experience can prepare them for future endings in life. Endings in which one must say goodbye and then move on are seldom easy.

Sometimes members leave the group abruptly, and the other participants have fantasies about the reason for the sudden departure. When this happens, it is best to be honest about the reasons for departure and help the remaining members manage the feelings that result.

During closure or termination in the group, it is useless to begin a new activity or discussion, or to set new goals. The group task is completed. The discussion should bring closure to the group experience and support the participant's movement into the community or on to other tasks in life.

Some groups get closure, or work through termination, through specific activities. The last group meeting in a series might become a festive occassion with a party to send the participants off with a celebration to remember. Another way is to have refreshments and have participants pair off for private goodbyes. In some groups that we have led, patients made cards with well wishes for the departing members. These cards served as reminders of the accomplishments and fellowship that participants experienced.

Regardless of how closure is managed, it is important for the leader to be sensitive to the participants' need to bring an end to the group experience and to allow time for this process to occur.

New Beginnings

In chapter 2, we proposed that in system theory the outcome of a group could be thought of as not just a time for ending, but as a time for new beginnings. As we conclude our discussion of outcome, we emphasize this again. What each participant, leader included, takes from the group becomes a part of who they are, and goes with them into their future interactions. The leader may look back on the group's development, and in retrospect, see places where he or she would like to try something different the next time a similar activity group is conducted. Patient members, too, may have gained confidence, acquired new information, or learned specific skills (so-called "outcomes") that will cycle into the next group in which they participate.

At best, the concept of endings and beginnings is an arbitrary but convenient way to talk about life experiences. In reality, it may not be possible to state where a group experience ends except in the strictest temporal sense. Psychological, cognitive, spiritual, social, and physical effects ripple out as from a stone cast into the water, influenced by all that exists within the boundaries of the shore. Such is the nature of all systems.

PART II

11
Group Protocol

The planning and preparation that occurs before the therapeutic activity group meeting is important for a successful group outcome. The leader's planning and preparation may be presented in a written format, called a *group protocol.* In the literature there are multiple formats for the group protocol. The system viewpoint influences the format used to describe the groups in this section.

The group protocol includes the following: 1) a description of the rationale for establishing a particular activity group; 2) the purpose of the group or its goals; 3) the criteria for selecting group participants; 4) the structure of the activity group; 5) a description of the environment in which the group occurs; 6) a description of the materials needed for the therapeutic activity; 7) a delineation of the roles and responsibilities of the therapist-leader; 8) an outline of the session format; 9) the intended outcome of the activity group experience; and 10) specific leader strategies and/or activity variations which may be used to meet the needs of particular populations.

Therapist-leaders use protocols to plan treatment experiences that make optimum use of available resources, and that complement the other treatment components in the health care environment. The protocol is also used as a group plan, which the therapist uses as a guide when implementing the therapeutic activity group. This guide can serve as a resource for adapting the activity and problem solving during the group experience.

Twenty-three activity group protocols follow, provided as a resource for the reader.

Get Acquainted

Source

Jones, J. E., 1980. Autographs: An Ice Breaker. In *The 1980 Annual Handbook for Group Facilitators* (9th annual), ed. J. W. Pfeiffer and J. E. Jones. San Diego, CA: University Associates.

Description/Rationale

A warm-up or get-acquainted experience can help group participants feel more comfortable, and begin to establish feelings of ownership and cohesion, to support the accomplishment of group goals.

Group Goals

1. To provide a non-threatening environment for getting acquainted.
2. To facilitate group participant interaction and getting acquainted.
3. To get the participants actively involved in the first group meeting.

Selection Criteria

Participants should be oriented to time, place, and person.

Group Structure

Size: five members or more

Length of session: fifteen minutes to an hour depending on group size

Duration: one time, or at the first meeting of a group with new members

Environment

Area with work surface plus large enough area to allow participants to circulate and meet one another.

Materials

Paper and pencil, worksheets, blackboard or flip chart, and felt tip marker.

Leader's Role

Create autograph sheet.

Facilitate interaction.

Monitor the experience and change the pace as needed to complete the activity sequence.

Session Format

The leader introduces the group and states the goals of the experience.

Each participant is given a pencil and the worksheet, and is asked to complete it. Group members follow the instructions on the worksheet or the leader gives the following instructions:

"You are to stand up and walk around the room and mingle with the members of the group. On the paper I have given you, please get the autograph of those group members who were born in states other than Texas (leader's home state). You may sit down after you have at least five (or whatever number determined) autographs." Thus, members circulate, meet one another, and gain autographs during the time period (see figure 11.1 for sample worksheet that can be used)

Autograph Worksheet

Place an X in front of those items for which you wish to solicit an autograph. When you are finished look around the room and try to identify persons which may provide the signature for your checked items. Wait for leader to tell you when to circulate and ask for signatures

_____ Person who eats pizza for breakfast   _____

_____ Person who has a dog for a pet   _____

_____ Person who recently moved to here   _____

_____ Person who wants to be in this group   _____

_____ Person who likes to swim   _____

_____ Person born in 1944   _____

_____ Person who might find me attractive   _____

_____ Person recently divorced   _____

_____ Person who has three children   _____

_____ Person who drives a sports car   _____

_____ Person who likes him/herself

Note: The items on the autograph sheet may vary depending on the needs, interests, abilities and values of the participants and the focus of the group in which this warm-up exercise is used. The elements may have a humorous or serious nature. Therapists should design a worksheet that is compatible with the setting and group treatment system.

Figure 11.1   Autograph Worksheet

When the leader notices that most of the group members have the number of autographs that they need, he or she asks the group members to be seated.

When members are seated, the leader can lead a group discussion that recognizes the things that group members have in common (e.g., place of birth, interests, experiences, personal preferences, characteristics, etc.). The leader may choose to write specific categories on the blackboard (e.g., persons who like tennis, persons who live alone, persons who like to work with people, persons who like team sports, etc.), and then write the name of group members under the identified categories. If appropriate, the group could then pick the theme to discuss (e.g., living alone: benefits and frustrations, myths and realities) or the group leader could give a home-work assignment (e.g., Before the next group all those interested in tennis get together and talk about the location of your favorite courts, your most memorable game, or make arrangements for a match; or before the next group those that live alone get together and plan the agenda for our next meeting).

If this activity is a group warm-up, then the leader briefly identifies/ summarizes the things that group members have in common, and the next group experience is introduced.

Variations

Seek autographs of patients who are in private rooms, have been in the hospital for more than a week, have been in occupational or recreational therapy before; obtain as many autographs as possible; see if you can get to know a personal historical fact from each participant before you get his or her autograph (e.g., person's birth date. how long they've lived here, how many brothers and sisters they have).

Expected Outcome

Participants will experience a nonthreatening activity that will promote interaction and help them to get to know each other.

Special Strategies

None

Goal Setting During and After Treatment

Source

Dell Orto, A.E. and R.G. Lasky, 1979. *Group Counseling and Physical Disability.* North Scituate, MA: Duxbury Press, 381.

Description/Rationale

Following an injury or disabling illness, people frequently need to review their present goals and evaluate the feasibility of these goals. A group-structured experience can be used by persons with physical disabilities to increase their awareness of goals in life and in treatment. The experiences are designed to help the participants to identify goal direction, and evaluate the goals' compatibility with his or her present (and future) life situation possibilities.

Group Goals

1. Participant will identify one or more goals in each of the following areas: life, treatment, and group.
2. If the participant has multiple goals, he or she will prioritize the goals.
3. Participant will be assisted in refining goal statements in order to make them achievable.
4. Participant will share goals with group members.
5. Participant will select one to three goals, and identify the possible ways to pursue these goals, either through the group or in the community.

Selection Criteria

Persons receiving treatment for disabling physical problems. (Note: We feel that goal setting is an activity applicable to many treatment settings and recommend this format for other populations besides those that have a physical disability.) Persons who lack direction or are unable to state their goals. Persons who may be able to identify their problems or desires but are not able to articulate them as goals.

Group Structure

Size: five to eight patients

Length of session: two hours

Duration: one time session, may be used at the beginning as well as when terminating treatment

Environment

In- or outpatient setting, treatment or prevention focus.

Writing surface (table or clipboard).

Comfortable room, movable chairs (circle placement to facilitate discussion).

Materials

Paper and pencils, felt tip pens, flip chart or blackboard.

Leader's Role

Prepare group introduction and goals worksheet.

Introduce group.

Structure and monitor activity.

Facilitate discussion and feedback.

Session Format

Group introduction (or lecturette which summarizes the ways to determine goals [e.g., through identifying problems, making wishes, focusing on key areas of life etc.]).

During a five to ten minute period, group members write their personal goals for life, treatment and in the group, identifying separate categories for each. A specific number of goals may be suggested.

Next, during a round robin discussion, each patient shares one or more of his or her goals in the category identified by the leader.

Following the goal sharing, the leader facilitates a discussion of the similarities and differences among the goals shared, and may note these on a blackboard or flip chart.

The leader then suggests that the members review their goals privately and prioritize the goals; if members need assistance in setting priorities, the group may be divided into pairs, and partners can assist in prioritization. Some leaders choose to set priorities from most to least important or vice-versa.

Members then share their first priority in one or more categories (treatment, life, group) and the leader will listen for a theme that emerges from among the participants and relate this theme to a possible group focus or future group activities. If goals can not be pursued in the group, the leader facilitates a discussion of other resources for goal pursuit.

Group ends with members' completing a written statement that identifies one goal that each participant will work on during the next week, month, or any specified time period.

Expected Outcome

Participants will have shared common experiences that relate to having a disability, have identified a specific focus for treatment and have experienced support from group peers for their goal pursuits

Variation

Prior to writing goals, each group member would complete a goals checklist. The list includes items related to specific goal themes; disability goals, achievement goals, personality change goals, and functional performance goals (see Figure 11.2).

Problem	Goals in Life	Goals for Treatment	Group Goal

Goal(s):_____

_____

_____

Figure 11.2   Goal Worksheet

Day Care Activity Group

Source

Howe, M., 1968. An occupational therapy activity group. *American Journal of Occupational Therapy*, 22(3):176–179.

Description/Rationale

Some patients have a problem verbalizing in the therapeutic community groups, and could profit from an opportunity to express themselves and experience group interrelationships. The model of Slavson's activity group was used, although with some differences, since Slavson's model was designed for use with children. Changes come about not through insight or interpretation, but through participation in a group experience.

Group Goals

Patients will:

1. Exhibit changes in self-image.
2. Exhibit improved relationships with peers and those in authority.
3. Show increased ability to respond to emotional issues.

Selection Criteria

Heterosexual group. Most participants were quiet or withdrawn, and judged "not profiting from other, insight-oriented groups." Patients tended to range from age fifteen to twenty-four. Participation was by prescription or at the patient's request.

Group Structure

Size: approximately eight patients (number fluctuated because this was an open group)

Length of session: one hour

Duration: group met two times per week, following the larger community group meeting; an open, ongoing group

Environment

A psychiatric day treatment center.

Leader's Role (co-lead by occupational therapist and psychiatric aide; one male, one female)

To participate in the activity.

To be supportive, responsive, nonjudgmental.

To structure and intervene if necessary.

Session Format

Each meeting is designed to be complete within itself and has three phases:

Planning Phase: Planning is left up to patients, with or without suggestions from the therapist.

Activity Phase: Spent in one of three ways:
(a) a sports activity at local park
(b) community field trip
(c) project at the day-care center

Evaluation Phase: Group comes back to day center lounge and discusses feelings about activity, the leader, the planning phase, etc. Participants are asked to complete a form anonymously, indicating whether or not the group session met their needs, plus any personal comments.

Expected Outcome

Patients will take more responsibility for themselves.

Patients will feel a part of the group.

Patients gain rudimentary skills in giving and receiving feedback.

Additional Information

Attendance was encouraged but not compulsory. The emphasis was on patients making choices and decisions. Decisions were made by consensus. Any new member was considered by the group, then *invited* to join. This increased the group's sense of power (though no potential participant was rejected).

Soap Opera Group

Source

Falk-Kessler, J. and K. Froschauer, 1978. The soap opera: A dynamic approach for psychiatric patients. *American Journal of Occupational Therapy,* 32(5):317–319.

See also:
Kilguss, A., 1977. The therapeutic use of a soap opera discussion group with psychiatric inpatients. *Clin. Social Work,* 5:58–65.

Description/Rationale

It was found that many chronic psychiatric patients watch a great deal of television in solitude during their leisure time. Television was chosen as the activity medium in order to decrease patients' resistance to the group experience. Soap operas were felt to have exaggerated, but familiar, life situations (p. 318) into which patients can project, and which would facilitate a discussion of personal experiences and problem solving experiences.

Group Goals

The participant will exhibit:
1. Increased attention and concentration.
2. Increased tolerance of others in the group.
3. Decreased inappropriate behaviors, such as inappropriate laughter.
4. Increased ability to retain information for use in problem solving.
5. Decreased social isolation.
6. Increased ability to acknowledge and express feeling and affect.
7. Increased ability to accurately assess the feelings of others.

Selection Criteria

All psychiatric patients at this day treatment center were included, including those initially psychotic.

Group Structure

Size: ten to fifteen patients

Length of session: sixty minutes, two times per week

Duration: an average of four months

Materials

Television

Environment

Day treatment, psychiatric care.

Living room atmosphere, with television as focus initially, then a discussion arrangement created.

Leader's Role

Leaders (two are implied) watch television with the group and chat with them, emphasis being on role-modeling. During the discussion phase, role playing is used, and sometimes psychodrama techniques.

Session Format

First Phase: Patients and leaders watch a soap opera together.

Second Phase: A discussion follows which focuses on the events of the program that day. Members may be asked to project into the story and react to events, and to share their own experiences. Role playing and other psychodramatic techniques are used to aid in reality testing, emotional clarification, and to allow members to explore healthy alternatives for problem solving.

Expected Outcome

Social gains related to previously stated group goals.

Documentation

The authors felt that gains were evident, and that the soap opera did act as a catalyst, as hoped. However, because the group occurred within an overall inpatient treatment milieu, they felt that patient progress could not be specifically and directly correlated to the activity group.

Body-Ego Movement Group

Source

May, P., M. Wexler, J. Salkin, and T. Schoop, 1978. Nonverbal techniques in the re-establishment of body image and self identity: A report. In *Therapy in Motion*, ed. M. N. Costonis, 135–152. Urbana, IL: University of Illinois Press.

Description/Rationale

Body image refers to the composite picture we have of our own body, partly conscious, largely unconscious. Body image has been found to be disturbed in many seriously disturbed and regressed patients, including those considered to be schizophrenic.

A "body-ego technique" is used that was developed by dance therapists Salkin and Schoop. The focus is on "reactivating and recalling the lost physical memory traces of emotions, and some of the associated lost objects" (p. 142–143). This allows their reintegration into the self.

Group Goals

To normalize body image and thereby influence behavior.

Selection Criteria

Those considered to have body-image disturbance. In this study, chronic, regressed schizophrenics.

Group Structure

Size: not described (we recommend six to twelve patients)

Length of session: forty minutes, three times per week

Duration: six months

Materials

Not described.

Environment

Not described. (We recommend a room with little furniture, adequate space for patients to move and walk around; initially a circle of chairs with space in between them plus space for storing chairs when they are not needed.)

Leader's Role

To "educate," otherwise not specified. (We suggest that the leader be an active role model and participate in the gross motor activities; participation may be decreased as the patients' ability to participate increases.)

Session Format

Sessions are viewed as classes, with a deliberate educational/experiential focus. In beginning sessions, try to establish contact with participants through use of rhythms (e.g., clapping, hitting, stamping). Then, movements that accompany childhood emotions are taught (e.g., throwing, hitting, stroking, etc.). Patients are not asked to show feeling, but to imitate the movement.

In later sessions, patients may be asked to associate a specific action with a specific emotion or named person.

Over several sessions, patients are guided to experience the postures and movements associated with normal stages of infancy through adolescence.

Group Outcome

This group was part of a controlled group study. Following six months of group activity sessions, the participants were evaluated by means of projective batteries, psychological testing and independent rater observation. While no one was seen as "cured," improvement in several areas of affect and social behavior were consistently noted.

Poetry Therapy Group

Source

Crootof, C., 1985. Poetry therapy for psychoneurotics. In *Poetry as Healer: Mending the Troubled Mind*, ed. J. Leedy, 150–160. New York: Vanguard Press.

Description/Rationale

The author believes that while poems can be selected that correspond with patients' moods, the patient "can not be left in a morass of despondency from which the poet gives no indication of his ability to extricate himself." (p. 153) Therefore, poems are selected in which the poet expresses that he has suffered loss, despair, etc., but that he has pulled through. Poetry is a way for people to share and participate with others.

Group Goals

1. Patients respond to poems with their feelings and reactions.
2. Patients are accepting of each other.

Selection Criteria

Patients judged to be non-psychotic and with adequate functioning ego.

Group Structure

Size: eight to seventeen patients (participants may drift in during the session)

Length of session: not specified, but in accordance with a very informal atmosphere

Duration: not specified

Environment

Informal, simulating that of a living room.

Group was conducted at a mental health center.

Materials

Mimeo or copy equipment available for producing copies of poems.

Leader's Role

To read poem, usually copied and distributed.

To facilitate discussion.

Session Format

Not specified except that the leader brings the poem, distributes it, reads poems aloud, and asks for reactions.

It is stressed that the patients need not understand every line, although the leader can help to clarify the poem's intent where possible.

Expected Outcome

Patients become more involved with and accepting of each other. Patients gain hope that they will be able to handle their problems.

Role Conflict and Problem Solving

Source

Doyle, P., 1986. Roles: Understanding Sources of Stress. In *The 1986 Annual: Developing Human Resources*, eds. Pfeiffer and Goodstein. San Diego, CA: University Associates, 27–34.

Description/Rationale

A human relations group to promote discussion of roles and the stress that accompanies them, with a structured format for identifying role conflict and problem solving to minimize role stress.

Group Goals

1. Participants identify the roles they presently assume/fulfill.

2. Participants discuss the role stress/conflict that exists in their lives.

3. Participants share strategies for managing role stress and conflict.

Selection Criteria

Persons oriented to time, place, and persons with a general sense of boundaries.

Group Structure

Size: group of five to eight, or large group broken into three to five subgroups of four members each

Length of session: ninety minutes to two hours

Duration: one time or one of a series of groups with focus on problem solving, interpersonal relations or stress management

Environment

If one small group, a table with adequate space for each member to sit and write. If there are several subgroups, the room must be large enough for the participants to discuss the structured experience without disturbing one another.

Materials

Work sheet, pencil for each participant, newsprint flip chart and felt tip markers, or blackboard.

Leader's Role

Prepare mini-lecture that describes roles and how roles develop (or are absorbed) and influence daily life.

Prepare the role conflict worksheets.

Introduce group and give out worksheets.

Structure and monitor the activity and facilitate discussion and feedback.

Session Format

The group leader introduces the group and states the group's goals and the purpose of the structured role activity. The leader explains the meaning of life roles and gives examples of the roles that a person may assume.

Each participant is given a pencil and the role worksheet and is instructed to complete the worksheet. Each member should list at least four roles.

Allow approximately five to ten minutes to complete the sheet.

Ask each participant to share verbally the roles they assume and any characteristics that they noted. Sharing may occur in one small group or in subgroups if the group is large.

Then ask each member to write conflicts that exist as they fulfill their roles. Allow five to ten minutes. The written conflicts are then verbally shared with group members.

Ask each member to write at least one method that could reduce the role stress or conflict that he or she experiences. Allow five to ten minutes for this notation.

Then reassemble all members as one group (large or small) and solicit the role stresses/conflicts that exist. Also compile the participants' suggestions for reducing stress. The group leader writes these on the flip chart for all to see. The leader then facilitates a discussion of common types of role stress and conflict, strategies for reducing role stress and conflict. Twenty to thirty minutes is needed for discussion.

Expected Outcome

Participants will have a sense of the common roles, responsibilities, and stresses that they share, and will have ideas for managing the stresses that they experience.

Variation

The activity can be limited to work roles or other role category.

Special Strategies

Lecturette Sources: '76 Annual: "Interrole Exploration"; Available from University Associates, San Diego, CA.

Changing Personal Limitations into Strengths through Values Clarification

Source

Conversion of Limitations (p. 137–138). In Smith, M., 1977. *Value Clarification.* CA: University Associates Publishers and Consultants.

Description/Rationale

Sometimes patients have limitation which can not be changed. Therefore, they usually learn to accept or cope with their limits. In some instances, a personal limit can be changed into a positive characteristic (e.g., "I hate kids" could become "I prefer being with adults," or "I relate well with adults".) During this values clarification group, the participants identify their values and assign them personal attributes which will support their function in daily life.

Group Goals

1. Participant will identify his or her strengths and limitations within the context of specific life roles.

2. Participant will convert an identified personal limit into a positive valued personal characteristic (e.g., "I am afraid in large groups," becomes "I like having a few close friends.")

3. When participant is unable to convert a limit into a positive personal characteristic, he or she will identify alternatives to develop the personal strengths desired.

4. Participant will help peers convert limitations to strengths or positive personal characteristics, or assist peers in identifying strategies to remedy limitations.

Selection Criteria

Patients oriented to time, place, and person, and with a sense of boundaries.

Those feeling overwhelmed by their problems and limitation and/or are re-evaluating their values and their values impact on daily life.

Group Structure

Size: eight to twelve participants

Length of session: sixty to ninety minutes

Duration: one-time meetings, or one of a series of groups that focus on self-image or life skills

Environment

In- or outpatient setting, treatment or prevention situation.

Writing surface (table or clipboard), circle of chairs for discussion and feedback session.

Materials

Worksheet (or paper), pencils, blackboard/flip chart, and felt tip markers.

Worksheet description: Divide a piece of typing paper into four columns: Title column 1 *Strengths*, column 2 *Limitations*, column 3 *Underlying Values*, and column 4 *Converted Characteristic* (see Figure II.4a and Figure II.4b)

Leader's Role

Prepare conversion worksheet.

Introduce group with description of roles and their attributes and the values that underlie these attributes.

Give worksheet.

Structure and monitor activity.

Facilitate discussion and feedback.

Session Format

The leader gives a brief introduction regarding the roles that one can have in life (parent, spouse, friend, worker) and gives examples of characteristics of these roles.

Subject: Life's Roles	Present	Feelings About	Locus of Control	Desired

Figure 11.3a Life Roles

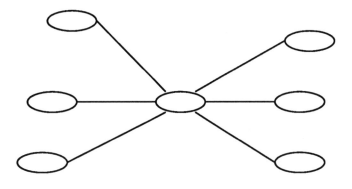

Roles	Conflict Characteristics

Possible Conflict Solutions			

Figure 11.3b   Roles Worksheet

The group participants are then given five to ten minutes to write their roles, and the strengths or limitations that they feel they have in fulfilling these roles.

The leader then facilitates a discussion of the strengths each person has identified. After each patient has shared his or her strengths, the leader facilitates the sharing of limitations and asks the group members to help each of their peers convert a limitation into a positive personal characteristic. For example, person is unable to repair their own car and hates being dependent on automobile mechanics. The underlying positive value is the person's desire to be in control of situations and to have increased knowledge and skills.

Next suggest that members share (in pairs) ideas for gaining the knowledge and skills required to facilitate the change from a limitation to a positive personal characteristic.

If time permits and patient attention endures —

After each member has had an opportunity to convert a limitation into a personal strength, the group leader may then pursue a brainstorming session to identify the means to achieve the change from limitation to personal strength.

If there is a series of values groups, the patients may be requested to keep a values journal.

Subject: Life's Roles	Present	Feelings About	Locus of Control	Desired
Friend		Feel lonely		Would like to have friends
Student	Go to school full time		No control over my schedule	
Lover	Just broke up with my boyfriend		His choice	Want to be appreciated
Worker	Part-time	Not make enough money		
Patient		Suicide was the only choice		Get out of here as quick as I can

Figure 11.3c   Sample Patient Worksheet: Life Roles

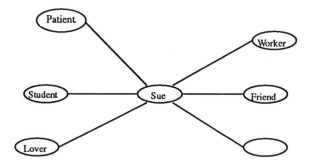

Roles	Conflict Characteristics
Student	Poor grades; not enough time to study.
Lover	He found somebody he liked better.
Friend	I don't have time for friends nor for fun.
Worker	My boss always needs me to work overtime.
Patient	I don't want to be seen as crazy Staff always tell me what to do.

Possible Conflict Solutions			
Student	Worker	Friend/Lover	Patient
Get a tutor Schedule your study time Go to "learn to study class"	Tell your boss no Look for a new job	Schedule time for friends Join a church group to meet people. Join a health club Talk to neighbors	Talk to staff about wanting more responsibility Ask doctor to give off grounds privileges

Note: After looking at these responses, the therapist might suggest that the patient establish a daily schedule to better organize her time and manage the stress of too much to do and too little time. Or patient could benefit from role playing situations in which she asks authority figures to consider her needs rather than being compliant and stressed due to anger or overcommitment.

Figure 11.3d   Sample Patient Roles Worksheet

Expected Outcome

Participants will have a review of their personal strengths and limitations, a general idea of the underlying values of their role attributes, and alternative methods for utilizing their strengths.

Variation

If group members are capable of working in subgroups, four or five patients may help each other complete the form and brainstorm for ideas to achieve the changes desired. Subgroups would then come together in a large group to share their subgroup experience and their ideas for changing limitations into positive characteristics.

Special Strategies

None

Role	Talents	Limitations	Conversion
Conversion = Restatement of a limitation as a positive value.			

Figure 11.4a   Conversion of a Limits to Strengths

Role	Talents	Limitations	Conversion
Worker	Dedicated Conscientious Skilled	Not social with my peers Won't attend advanced workshop to learn something new	Prefer friendships outside of work Like doing work routines that don't change;
Roommate	Good friend Good cook I like to help others Good listener	Hate to put my things away I'm disorganized I procrastinate	I always meet my deadlines
		Conversion = Restatement of a limitation as a positive value.	

Figure 11.4b   Conversion of Limits to Strengths: Patient Example

Self-Image Collage

Source

Morris, I. T. and K. M. Cinnamon, 1975. *A Handbook of Non-verbal Group Exercises*. Springfield, IL: Charles C. Thomas Publisher.

Description/Rationale

As we grow and change throughout life, we develop, redefine and refine our self-image. Given the illnesses and crises that patients have experienced and the problems that result, most patients can benefit from reviewing their image and getting feedback from others about their presentation of self.

Group Goals

Participants will identify values, attitudes, characteristics, behaviors, and roles that make up one's self-image.

Each participant will complete a paper bag collage that reflects his or her self-image.

Participants will share his or her view of him or herself with each other.

Participants will give feedback to each other about their self-image.

Selection Criteria

Persons who are oriented to time, place, and person. They have boundaries, but a weakened sense of self due to a developmental transition, accident, injury, or illness.

Group Structure

Size: even number of participants (eight to sixteen)

Length of session: sixty minutes, (longer if the group is large)

Duration: one session, could be a module of a series of self-image or interpersonal communication groups)

Environment

In- or outpatient setting, health care or prevention setting.

Work surface for collage making.

Circle seating arrangement for discussion.

Materials

Various types of magazines that are compatible with the interests of the participants, scissors, glue, and brown paper bags.

Leader's Role

Introduce group and describe its purpose.

Monitor the activity work period (collage making) and help participants as needed.

Structure the discussion and feedback session.

Session Format

Introduce the group members.

Introduce the group and its goals and give a few brief comments regarding one's self-image (physical appearance, values, attitudes, goals, interests, personal characteristics, [such as happy, shy, persuasive] etc.)

Give each participant a brown paper bag and let the participants construct their self-image collage. You may use pictures, words, phrases, or any combination of these. Usually a collage can be completed in about twenty minutes.

Divide the group into pairs. Ask one person of the pair to put the paper bag collage on his or her head and wear it for a few minutes. Ask the other person to study his or her partner's self-image collage for about two to three minutes, and then to remove the bag from the partner's head. Next, he or she should share how they view them after looking at the collage. The collage wearer then has the opportunity to give feedback to the partner, and to state whether the observations are accurate of whomever the person sees, or if the person sees him or herself differently, describing some of these differences.

The partners then switch roles and the previous observation, sharing, and feedback session is repeated.

The participants then rejoin each other in one large group and have an opportunity to share what they learned about their self-image (from the experience, the interpretation, or the feedback), or what they learned about their partner, and also to share what they felt about the therapeutic activity group.

Expected Outcome

Participants will review, reaffirm, and identify the roles that contribute to their self-image, and the personal values and attitudes that support these roles. Participants will share their knowledge and attitudes with a peer and get feedback from the other group participants.

Special Strategies

The collage experience can be varied, for example, present roles may be depicted on the outside of the bag, and roles desired in the future on the inside. Physical characteristics and interests may be depicted on the outside, and values and attitudes on the inside of the bag. The focus of discussion can also be varied.

The collage experience could also have a group image focus rather than an individual image focus. Each group member is requested to depict the group on the outside of the bag, and attitudes, values, and interests that support this image on the inside. During the discussion the group identity is discussed: varied views of the image, changes desired, specifics related to values and attitudes, and other interests.

Social Network (Interpersonal Skills) Group

Source

Stroud, M. and E. Sutton, 1988. *Activities Handbook and Instructor's Guide for Expanding Options for Older Adults with Developmental Disabilities.* Baltimore: Paul Brookes Publishing.

Description/Rationale

Many people undergoing treatment in mental health settings have an interest in or a need to improve their interpersonal skills. The basis of skill development is an understanding of the individual's social network, who is included in this network, and how these persons influence the individual. One component of the social system includes the individual's affective relationships, including romantic, friendship, parental, and spouse relationships. Once the benefits and stresses of these relationships are understood, the group participant can decide which social skills need refinement and identify methods for managing the relationship stresses that may be present.

Group Goals

1. To identify the affective relationships in one's social network.
2. To identify the benefits of affective relationships.
3. To identify the stresses of affective relationships.
4. To identify the contributions that one makes to an affective relationship.
5. To identify methods of managing stresses of an affective relationship.

Selection Criteria

Persons oriented to time, place, and person, and who have a sense of their boundaries.

Youth through older adult age groups of people who need to evaluate, redefine, or develop affective relationships.

Members of a "significant other" support group; such as those attended by citizens with developmental disabilities, abused spouses, parents of learning-disabled children, families of Alzheimer's disease victims, and so on. These "significant others" provide a major support to patients who have a chronic illness or disability and can benefit from discussing the stresses of these affective relationships and from joint problem-solving for managing these stresses.

Group Structure

Size: five to twelve patients or "significant others"

Length of session: sixty to ninety minutes

Duration: one time, or a part of a series of groups with self-image, communication or interpersonal relations focus

Materials

Paper and pencils, worksheet (social network, see figure, Social Network), blackboard/flip chart and felt tip markers.

Leader's Role

Prepare brief introduction to define and exemplify one's social network.

Prepare and distribute social network worksheet.

Structure and monitor activity.

Facilitate discussion and feedback.

Session Format

Statement of group goals.

Brief lecturette defining social network and affective relationships and give examples (e.g., love from parents, siblings, friends, romances, marriage; love for children, pets, etc.) friendships in the community, at work or in the neighborhood.

During a five to ten minute period ask participants to list five or more affective relationships that they have experienced. After listing the relationship, also list names of the persons in this relationship; (e.g., love from siblings — Tom and Michelle, friends at work — Harry and Jim, etc.).

Alternative — Ask participants to complete the social network diagram. Each person writes his or her name in the middle circle and then puts identified affective relationships in the surrounding circles. The names of the significant others of the affective relationship are written by the surrounding circles. (See Figure 11.5a for an example.)

Hold a brainstorming session (five to ten minute) or divide the group in pairs and ask the participants to identify the benefits of affective relationships. List the contributions from the pairs or during the brainstorming on the blackboard or flip chart.

During the next five to ten minute period identify and list the stresses.

Provide a brainstorming period (ten to fifteen minutes) to elicit methods for managing stresses in affective relationships (e.g., asking friends or family for help when you need it, have the group identify the supports in the community, [paid or unpaid] if they have few in the family or at work, etc.).

Have participants list the ways in which they contribute to affective relationships; ways in which they show/express affection (e.g., helping spouse at home, taking child to movie, offering to give a co-worker a ride to work when his or her auto is not working, etc.).

Use round robin discussion format to allow each participant to share his or her contributions to affective relationships.

Group summary

Reiterate groups goals.

Summarize what was learned in the group (mutual participant and leader summary).

Identify directions for future groups (e.g., learning to share oneself with others in affective relationships, identifying one's support network and learning to use it).

Variations

The use of brainstorming varies with participant ability.

If participants are unable to complete the individual worksheets, the leader can focus more generally on what is a social network and make one drawing on the blackboard (similar to that in the social network diagram) and lead a discussion in which group participants give suggestions that define one's social network. (See Figures 11.5a amd 11.5b.)

Expected Outcome

Participants will know what a social network is, be able to define their role in it and understand how the network influences their interpersonal skills and life stress. Participants will also identify the ways in which they can contribute to affective relationships.

Special Strategies

None

Friendship, Making Friends

Source

Merritt, R. E. and D. D. Walley, 1977. *The Group Leader's Handbook: Resources, Techniques, and Survival Skills.* Champaign, IL: Research Press Co.

Description/Rationale

Frequently patients feel lonely, isolated, and that they have few friends. Sometimes they feel that they have little to contribute in a friendship, and thus they avoid pursuing interpersonal relationships. In a group, participants can learn about and experience friendship and get feedback from participants about their personal attributes which make up friendship.

Group Goals

1. Participants will identify the characteristics of a friend.
2. Participants will identify their personal characteristics which make them a good friend.
3. Participants will determine interest in making new friendships.
4. Participants will discuss and share strategies for making new friends.

Selection Criteria

Persons oriented to time, place, and person, and having a sense of boundaries. Those who are dissatisfied with peer relationships and/or want to establish a social network.

Group Structure

Size: eight to sixteen people

Length of session: sixty minutes (longer for a larger group)

Duration: a one-time meeting or part of a series of groups that focuses on roles and interpersonal relationships.

Environment

In- or outpatient setting.

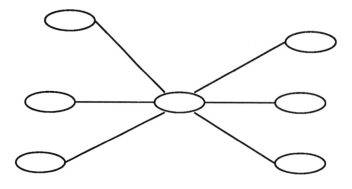

Relationships:	My Contributions

Relationship:	
Benefits	**Stresses**

Figure 11.5a Social Network

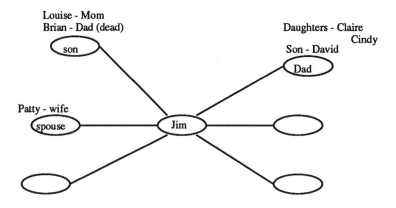

Relationships:	My Contributions
Husband	Earn a good living. Faithful to my wife.
Father	Love my kids. Buy nice clothes, pay for school.
Son	Mother lives with us since her stroke six months ago.

Relationship: Son	
Benefits	**Stresses**
Minimize cost for the care of my mother. I am helping my mother as my father would if he were alive. My children have an opportunity for a close relationship with their grandmother.	Family feels that she should be in a nursing home. We worry about leaving her home alone if we go out as a family. My wife feels the extra stress from an additional person to care for.

Figure 11.5b   Social Network: Patient Example

Treatment or prevention situation.

Writing surface (table or clipboard).

Circle of chairs for discussion and feedback.

Materials

Worksheet (or paper), pencils, newsprint flip chart and felt tip markers, or blackboard.

Leader's Role

Prepare friendship worksheets.

Introduce group with description of friendship (or read a poem or short essay that describes friendship).

Give worksheets and pencils.

Structure and monitor the activity.

Facilitate dicussion and feedback.

Session Format

Introduction of group members.

Group leader introduces the group, states the goals for participation.

Group leader may give mini-lecture regarding friendship qualities or characteristics, or could read friendship poem.

Participants complete the mini worksheet "Friendship." (See figure 11.6.)

Large group discussion of characteristics of a friend — list on the blackboard or the flip chart.

Participants then complete the worksheet section in which they identify their own characteristics as a friend.

Participants are then divided into pairs and share their own characteristics as a friend with their partner.

Participants come together again in a large group and the partners introduce each other to the rest of the group. For example, if Bill and Elizabeth have been partners, leader says, "Bill, tell the group the characteristics that Elizabeth has shared with you as you introduce her to the group." He says, "This is my partner, Elizabeth, who likes to help friends when they are having trouble. They like her because she can keep her sense of humor when she is stressed. She'd like to help kids through the Big Sister program." Then Elizabeth introduces Bill, "This is my partner, Bill. He likes to get together with friends to watch football and drink beer. He doesn't know what he has to offer to friends...would like a girlfriend. . . ."

Leader gives each member an opportunity to add to their list of personal characteristics as a friend. Leader may need to add examples; prepare a few before the meeting in case you need them.

Leader reflects/summarizes the friendship characteristics and activities in which friendship was described and then asks the large group to share the ideas they have for how to pursue friendship. These ideas are recorded on the blackboard or flip chart for all to see.

Leader then asks the participants to record on the Friendship worksheet an activity they wish to pursue to develop a friendship.

Expected Outcome

Participants are optimistic about their possible role as a friend and they can identify potential resources for establishing friendships.

Special Strategies

A lecturette source: Carnegie, D. and A. Pell, 1981. *How to Win Friends and Influence People* (Revised for the 80s). New York: Pocket Books.

Participants could be given assignments and make commitments in written contracts.

Assertiveness Group

Source

Bruce, M., and B. Borg, 1987. *Frames of Reference in Psychosocial Occupational Therapy*. Thorofare, NJ: Slack, Inc.

Description/Rationale

Individuals who can't set limits on others, nor ask for what they need, often end up angry and/or depressed. These persons may profit by gaining "permission for" and practice with making their needs known. The group role-play format has historically proven a useful vehicle for providing such practice.

Friendship Worksheet

Name: _____

Names of two or more friends: _____

_____

What do you like about these friends:

_____

_____

_____

Three or more activities you share with friends:

_____

_____

_____

How frequently do you see your friends?

_____

How do you usually go about making friends?

_____

_____

What keeps a friendship going?

_____

_____

My personal characteristics that make me a good friend:

_____

_____

Figure 11.6 Friendship

Group Goals

Participants will gain skills needed to:

1. Ask for what they desire.

2. Say "no," or otherwise set appropriate limits.

3. Identify socially acceptable alternatives for responding in common social situations.

Selection Criteria

Persons who have difficulty asking for what they want, who feel "pushed around," who are overly apologetic, who lack confidence with the give-and-take of common social exchange.

Group Structure

Size: five to eight participants

Length of session: forty minutes to one hour, depending on members' tolerance

Duration: twice a week, four or five weeks (typically eight to ten sessions)

Environment

In- or outpatient setting; health care or prevention situation.

Comfortable room, movable seating, enough room for several people to stand and move about.

Materials

Dependent on context of role plays. Leader may desire blackboard or large paper to highlight concept before or after role plays.

Leader's Role (Co-leaders are helpful)

To describe the group's purpose.

To provide initial didactic information pertaining to assertive behavior.

To get participants' suggestions regarding role-play situations.

To set the stage for role plays selected.

To act as an alter-ego, or help prompt individual participants if they need assistance.

To model effective responses, if needed.

To record goals and progress.

Session Format

In the first session, the leader asks participants to list (in order of least to most difficult) five social situations in which they feel unable to make their needs known. The leader looks for common features in the lists, then creates a hierarchy of situations that will be used for the group's role plays.

If desired, didactic information is given regarding assertive behavior, the difference between assertiveness and aggressiveness, and so on.

In each session, one or more situations is acted out. The situations are enacted in order from least to most difficult, with participants taking turns playing a variety of roles, being both the "giver" and the "recipient" of appropriate assertiveness. The therapist may prompt, coach, and encourage, or may interrupt to model.

After the simulation, participants are asked to give each other verbal feedback.

As the group session nears completion, each participant identifies a specific assertive behavior he or she will attempt before the next meeting. Time is allowed at subsequent meetings for participants to state whether or not they achieved their goals.

Outcome

Participants will know the difference between assertive and aggressive behavior, practice assertive behaviors, and describe the various contexts in which assertive behavior is required.

Variations

Some leaders choose to introduce a relaxation exercise before the simulation begins or at its conclusion.

Video-taping of role plays is not uncommon, with the tape viewed by the participants used as a means to "critique" the effectiveness of given responses.

Time Management

Source

Dougherty, P. M. and M. Vining Radomski, 1987. *The Cognitive Rehabilitation Work Book.* Maryland: Aspen Publication.

Description/Rationale

A structured group experience designed to help patients identify their use of time and their weekly activities; evaluate their use of time; and provide support for planning a weekly schedule.

Group Goals

1. Each participant will complete a weekly activity checklist.
2. Each participant will identify the activities which need to be scheduled.
3. Each participant will identify and discuss the time conflicts that exist in his or her schedule.
4. Each participant will complete a hypothetical schedule for a given problem.
5. Each participant will plan a personal schedule for one week and evaluate his or her ability to follow the schedule.

Selection Criteria

Person who needs assistance with time management.

Group Structure

Size: five to ten patients, outpatients

Length of session: sixty minutes

Duration: one time, or a part of a series in daily living or self-management skills

Environment

Outpatient setting, health care or prevention setting.

Work surface (table or clipboards).

Room free of distraction, circle seating arrangement for discussion.

Materials

Paper and pencils, worksheets, flip chart and felt tip pen, or blackboard.

Leader's Role

Introduce concepts of time management.

Present worksheet.

Lead and monitor discussion, facilitate feedback among participants.

```
┌─────────────────────────────────┐
│        Activity Check List       │
│  Place an X in on the line in front │
│  of those activities in which you   │
│  frequently participate.            │
│  Daily Living Activities:           │
│  _____ Prepare breakfast            │
│                                     │
│  _____ Prepare dinner               │
│                                     │
│  _____ Do laundry                   │
│                                     │
│  _____ Clean apartment              │
│                                     │
│  _____ Maintain car                 │
│                                     │
│                                     │
│  Leisure Activities:                │
│  _____ Watch television             │
│                                     │
│  _____ Visit a friend               │
│                                     │
│  _____ Go to church                 │
│                                     │
│  Work Activities                    │
│                                     │
│  _____ Go to work                   │
│                                     │
└─────────────────────────────────┘
```

Note: This list is not comprehensive.

	Sun	Mon	Tues	Wed	Thurs	Fri	Sat	Comments
8:00								
9:00								
10:00								
11:00								
12:00								
1:00								

Source Adapted from Dougherty, P. M., and M. V. Radomski, 1987. *The Cognitive Rehabilitation Workbook,* Rockville, MD: Aspen, 281.

Figure 11.7a   Activity Checklist and Time Management Schedule

```
┌─────────────────────────────────┐
│        Activity Check List      │
│  Place an X in on the line in front │
│  of those activities in which you   │
│  frequently participate.            │
│                                     │
│  Daily Living Activities:           │
│  _____ Prepare breakfast           │
│                                     │
│    X   Prepare dinner               │
│  ____                               │
│                                     │
│  _____ Do laundry                  │
│                                     │
│    X   Clean apartment              │
│  ____                               │
│                                     │
│  _____ Maintain car                │
│                                     │
│  Leisure Activities:                │
│                                     │
│    X   Watch television             │
│  ____                               │
│                                     │
│  _____ Visit a friend              │
│                                     │
│  _____ Go to church                │
│                                     │
│  Work Activities                    │
│                                     │
│    X   Go to work                   │
│  ____                               │
└─────────────────────────────────┘
```

Note: This list is not comprehensive.

	Sun	Mon	Tue	Wed	Thurs	Fri	Sat	Comments
8:00		Tele-vision	———	———	———	——►		Mother does laundry
9:00		Work	Work	Work	Work	Work		Would like to get back to going to church
10:00	Break-fast						Clean Apart-ment	Not enjoying work; frequently late
11:00								
12:00								In evening usually watches TV
1:00		▼	▼	▼	▼	▼	Super market	

Source Adapted from Dougherty, P. M., and M. V. Radomski, 1987. *The Cognitive Rehabilition Workbook,* Rockville, MD: Aspen, 281.

Figure 11.7b   Sample Worksheet

Session Format

Leader introduces the group, describing time management and the goals of the experience.

During ten to fifteen minute period, each participant completes the weekly activity checklist.

Patients then share a summary of the activities that they do during a typical week.

Patients are asked to complete a schedule of activities that they have identified. (See figure 11.7a and figure 11.7b)

Depending upon patient ability, participants need ten to twenty minutes to complete this schedule.

Patients pair off and share their schedule with their partner.

Paired sharing is followed by a large group discussion in which patients can identify factors that cause time conflicts, stress, and concerns regarding following the schedule during the next week (keeping up with it). Discussion can also include strategies for managing conflicts, stress, or following schedule.

The group leader then gives this homework assignment: Take your completed calendar, tape it to your refrigerator (or door of the patient's room), and circle those scheduled items that you actually do. Also note any conflict or stresses that you experience. Each member then makes a commitment to follow his or her schedule for the upcoming week and agrees to report back to the group.

Therapist closes the group by reiterating the group goals, what has been learned in the group, and the benefits of time management.

Expected Outcome

Participants describe and monitor their use of time and evaluate how time management helps them to meet their responsibilities. They also have an opportunity to restructure their use of time and receive feedback about their ability to manage time effectively.

Special Strategies

Depending upon the patient's ability, the time schedule may include a week or a typical day or a sample of one or two days (e.g., workday and weekend day).

Time and Money Management

Source

Value Indicators: Time/Money. In Smith, M., 1977. *Value Clarification.* La Jolla, CA: University Associates.

Description/Rationale

Quality of life and daily life satisfaction are influenced by one's resources. The efficient use of time and money can improve one's performance in daily life as well as improve one's satisfaction. This values clarification group can help participants use time and money efficiently.

Group Goals

1. Participant will identify the ways in which he or she uses time and the way he or she spends money.
2. Based upon the participant's use of time and money, he or she will identify personal values related to the use of time and money.
3. Based upon the identification of values and estimated expenditures of time and money, the participant will determine if a change in these patterns is needed.
4. If change is desired, the person will determine the strategies needed to determine the use of time and money.

Selection Criteria

Person oriented to time, place, and person, with a sense of boundaries and dissatisfied with their time and money management skills.

Group Structure

Size: eight to twelve patients

Length of session: sixty to ninety minutes

Duration: one time, or one of a series of values clarification or daily living skill groups

Environment

In- or outpatient focus, treatment or prevention setting.

Writing surface (table or clipboard).

Movable chairs (form a circle to promote group boundaries and facilitate communication).

Weekly Activity Time Sheet				
Activity	**Time Spent per Week**	**Rank Order of Importance**	**Preferred Order**	**Related Value**
Work Prepare Perform Wind Down				
Family Spouse Children Parents Relatives				
Recreation Self Spouse Children Active Passive				
Self Self Care Sleep Rest				
Community Church School Political Other				

Desired Changes: _____

_____

_____

Figure 11.8a   Time and Values

Weekly Money Work Sheet				
Money Category	Money Spent per Week	Rank Order of Importance	Preferred Order	Related Value
Basic Food Shelter Clothes Transportation				
Work Travel Entertainment Dues Other				
Recreation Self Spouse Children Entertainment Vacation				
Future Saving investment Large purchase				
Other Church School Political Other				

Desired Changes: _____

_____

_____

Figure 11.8b   Money and Values

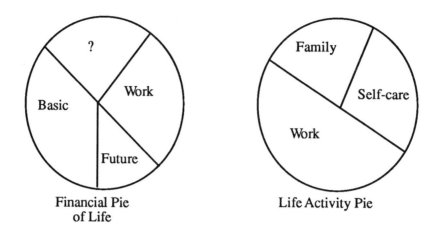

Financial Pie
of Life

Life Activity Pie

Figure 11.8c   Pie of Life (Financial / Activity)

Materials

Paper (or worksheet), pencils, blackboard or flip chart with felt tip markers.

Leader's Role

Prepare worksheets.

Introduce group.

Distribute worksheets.

Structure and monitor activity.

Facilitate discussion and feedback.

Session Format

The group leader gives a brief description of the group activity and discusses the relationship between one's values and the use of time as well as the influence of values upon one's financial management. Participants are reminded that work time includes travel, planning, and worrying about work, as well as time spent recuperating from work. A person must have the energy to invest in leisure before he can enjoy it. In other words, "a person who comes home from work and watches television is likely to be recuperating from work rather than indulging in recreation" (p. 124).

The group members are asked to reflect upon what they do during a typical week. On a flip chart, the leader writes the activities that participants share (e.g., work, family, recreation, and cultural activities). Following this warm-up, participants do the following activity:

Each group member completes an activities calendar worksheet or draws a pie-of-life that identifies the activities to which they devote time. Another worksheet or pie is then completed to identify the activities on which they spend financial resources.

Each of the sets of activities should then be rank-ordered, placing those which are of most importance first, and so on; or placing those which are most costly first, and so on.

Participants then share with other group members a summary of how they use time and money, and relate their use to the values that the participants hold.

Following the sharing, participants are then asked to note on their worksheets any changes that they wish to make in the use of their time or financial resources.

Strategies for making time and resource utilization changes may be done during the following group or during this group meeting if time allows. (See figures 11.8a, b, and c.)

Expected Outcome

Participants will understand the relationship between their values and the use of time and money. They will identify the manner in which they wish to use their time and money, and the restraints that influence their use.

Special Strategies

None

Community Cooking Group

Source

Bachner, S., 1987. Group Process in a Community Occupational Therapy Cooking Group. *In Group Process,* ed. M. Ross, 105—117, Thorofare, NJ: SLACK, Inc.

Description/Rationale

To be independent in the community, patients need daily living skills. Mastery of basic cooking principles not only helps participants meet their daily needs but supports their participation in one of the major social arenas of contemporary society. The community cooking group develops skills and supports independence and socialization. The six-session closed group considers physical, psycho-social, and cognitive abilities of the client/student. The group text is Bachner (1984) *Picture This: An Illustrated Guide to Complete Dinners.*

Group Goals

1. Student will master basic cooking skills: follow pictograph instructions, abide by safety and cleanliness standards, practice measurement of ingredients, and learn food substitutes.

2. Students will practice social skills and learn to work cooperatively with peers during meal preparation and clean-up.

3. Students will practice social skills during dinner and contribute to dinner conversation.

Selection Criteria

Adults with developmental disabilities who live in the community. (Note: We feel that patients who are making the transition to community living could also benefit from this model of treatment; a cookbook that meets the ability level of the participants would be used.)

Group Structure

Size: six students

Length of session: two hours, once a week

Duration: six sessions

Environment

Each group occurs in one of the student group members' homes. This allows the leaders to evaluate the environment to maximize learning and function in member's own kitchen. Since clients have developmental disabilities and may incur learning problems when trying to generalize skills, it is preferable to provide the learning experience in the actual environment in which they will perform (their own home or group residence).

Materials

Participant list, cookbook for each member, food. Participants pay $15.00 per session to cover the charges for staff and supplies.

Leader's Role (Co-leader required)

Allow for one leader for three students. (The supervision ratio could vary depending upon the abilities of the group participants.)

Session Format

Leader provides each member with the names and addresses of the participants to provide a resource for those who wish to car pool.

Introduction: Leader describes the six lessons in which members will learn basic cooking skills, have an opportunity to serve as host, and ultimately receive a certificate of completion.

Warm-up: Each session begins with a snack, hand washing and five to ten minute period of socialization.

The cooking session

The cooking tasks are delegated.

Food preparation ensues.

Table is set.

Meal served and eaten.

Clean up.

Session is reviewed, participant accomplishments recognized.

Expected Outcome

Participants will gain a reasonable level of competence in meal planning and preparation, enjoy an opportunity to socialize, and learn entertainment and host skills.

Special Strategies

The group model could be adapted to meet the needs of various levels of patient function. The concept could assist patients recently discharged who are adapting to community settings.

Documentation

Since this is a non-medical model group, documentation is not based upon the traditional SOAP format nor is it written for third party payers. Within a week of each cooking session, a note is sent to the student and/or "significant other." The note outlines the cooking session and the student's performance during the session. Notes do not use professional jargon but are written in lay terms. They should identify the strengths of the student's performance and suggest practice needed prior to the next cooking group.

Prevocational Group

Source

Kramer, L., 1984. *SCORE: Solving Community Obstacles and Restoring Employment.* New York: Haworth Press.

Description/Rationale

Before returning to work, participants may need to assess their work history, present employment needs, and present skill level. A prevocational group provides this opportunity and can prepare a person for a more successful job application interview.

Group Goals

1. Participant will share a summary of his or her work history.
2. Participant will identify the advantages and disadvantages of working.
3. Participant will identify present work interests and skill levels.
4. Participant will summarize work interests, skills, and history in a role play interview.

Selection Criteria

Adolescents through older adults who are oriented and boundaried and preparing to return to work.

Group Structure

Size: four to twelve participants

Length of session: sixty to ninety minutes

Duration: one time, one of fifteen educational modules during an eight-week period. Other groups include leisure assessment, job seeking process, interview skill practice, career objectives, and on-the-job communication skills.

Pre-vocational Screening

Name: _____

Please briefly describe the following:

Education history:

Employment history:

Last two jobs held:

Dates of employment (last two jobs):

Reason for leaving employment (last two jobs):

Employment application (in last two years):

Employment interviews (in last two years):

Present employment goal:

Other Possible Questions: Describe your present activity level; Satisfaction with activity level; Present goal at this time; Reason for attending group

---

Figure 11.9a Prevocational Screening Form. Adapted from Kramer, 1984 SCORE Haworth Press.

Environment

In- or outpatient setting.

Work surface for completing forms (table or clipboard).

Circle of chairs for discussion and role play experience.

Materials

Paper (prevocational forms), pencils, blackboard or flip chart.

Work Skills Checklist

Please place a check beside those items in which you
have had paid (or volunteer) experience.

Stocking shelves   ———

Cashiering   ———

Supervising others   ———

Driving a vehicle   ———

Host/Hostessing in a
Restaurant   ———

Waiter/Waitressing   ———

Other Skills Listed: Selling, Assembling Items in Factory, Repairing
Home, Typing, Telephone Answering, Counseling, Dishwashing,
Loading a Truck, Cooking/Baking, Office Machine Operating,
Teaching, Mail Room Sorting, Busing in a Restaurant, Building
Construction, Woodworking, Farming, Bookkeeping, Commercial
Painting, Auto Repairing, Housekeeping, Other.

Figure 11.9b   Work Skills Checklist Form. Adapted from
Kramer, (1984) SCORE.

Leader's Role

Develop worksheets.

Introduce group.

Present worksheets.

Monitor activity and structure it as needed.

Facilitate discussion and feedback.

Session Format

Leader introduces the group, talks about goals of the group, and
shares a few remarks about preparing for employment. For example, the
leader may review the value of work, the relationship of work with leisure,

Employment Opposing Forces	
Motivation to Work	**Barriers to Work**

Figure 11.9c Time and Values

the influence of work on self-care needs, and family and community roles. Preparation for employment may be outlined, identification of employment interests, assessment of work skills and formation of employment goals.

Following the introduction/lecturette, the participants complete the prevocational screening form (see figure 11.9a). Allow about ten minutes for completion.

After participants have completed the screening form, encourage each participant to summarize his or her employment history. (You could use a round robin strategy for this sharing.) Highlight any group themes that emerge, and summarize the importance of work history when applying for a job or returning to work.

Next ask the participants to complete the work skills checklist (see figure 11.9b). Allow about five minutes to do this. The leader may ask participants to share their present skill level based upon those identified on the completed checklist. This skill checklist may also be used to determine further assessment needs and individual treatment programs.

Participants are asked to complete the advantage/disadvantage worksheet (see figure 11.9c). This worksheet is then used to facilitate a group discussion which uses force field analysis to gain an understanding of the opposing forces that influence work/career choices, employment history, and job fulfillment.

Expected Outcome

Participants have adequate self-knowledge to describe their work history, skills, and interests to the group and are able to present this information in a role play interview.

Special Strategies

Group could focus on one particular employment category (e.g., working in a fast food restaurant, being a receptionist, factory worker, and so on

Reminiscence Group

Source

Authors (Borg, B. and M. A. Bruce)

Also see: Ingersoll, B. and L. Goodman, 1980. History becomes alive. Facilitating reminiscence in a group of institutionalized elderly. *Journal of Gerontological Social Work* 2(4):305–319.

Description/Rationale

Recalling and sharing with others regarding ones life experiences is a special way to keep those events real, to give something of oneself to others, and to integrate past experiences as one moves toward the future. Reminiscing is not only for older persons; it has a place for all of us, as we all experience life changes, putting events behind us, yet cherishing their significance to us. Reminiscence can evoke the strong feelings associated with personal experiences, including pleasure and satisfaction as well as dissatisfaction and grief at their loss. Recalled experiences can also serve as point of reference or provide a context for understanding and coping with new situations.

The group described has been used with older adults, but in principle (and with appropriate modification), could be used with persons of any age needing a chance for reflection.

Group Goals

1. To stimulate participants interest.

2. To provide a supportive environment for interpersonal sharing and reality testing.

3. To decrease feelings of isolation and anomie.

4. To create a context in which participants will be able to do the following:

   (a) Verbally share past experiences and present feelings.

   (b) Put present situations into a context based on personal history (i.e., discriminate differences and similarities between "then" and "now").

   (c) Give validation to the self and others in the group.

Selection Criteria

Older adults, persons experiencing change and/or loss, persons experiencing isolation.

Group Structure

Size: four to eight patients

Length of session: thirty-five to forty-five minutes, if participants can tolerate this time period

Duration: six to eight sessions

Environment

Casual, "homey" if possible

Materials

Depends on particular focus of the activity to be used in the sessions.

Old magazines, scissors, glue, personal photographs, etc.

Leader's Role

To facilitate interaction, especially to encourage a nonjudgmental climate.

To be a role model when possible.

To provide materials.

To monitor activity, provide assistance if needed.

Session Format

The leader helps with introductions, then describes briefly the purpose of the session(s) in a nonclinical way. Emphasis is on the opportunity participants have to share an enjoyable, memorable group experience.

The focus activity is described by the leader, and materials provided.

Sample focus activities include:

1. Leader (or participants, if asked in advance) brings old records to be listened to by the group (e.g., Big Band songs, songs associated with World War II, etc.). The group may be asked to try to guess artists, or to talk about where they were when these recordings were popular. Discussion may also focus on differences between

then and now. List of differences and similarities may be drawn up by the leader.

2. "Mom" or "Dad" collage: Participants are asked to make a collage that reflects their memories of their mother or father. These collages can be made in conjunction with celebrations for Mother's or Father's Day. Collages may be made of magazine pictures or freehand drawings.

3. Participants are asked ahead of time to bring to this session a favorite object given to them by someone else. They are asked to share with the group regarding the object and the giver's significance to them. (Leader may also bring in an object to talk about.)

4. Picture day: Participants are asked to bring a photograph of themselves taken many years ago (baby pictures or older). Members may try to guess who's who. Discussion focuses on the events going on in the person's life at the time of the photo. Contrasts may be drawn between then and now.

5. Grandma's trunk: A model truck or a symbolic representation of Grandma's trunk is placed in the center of the group. Participants are asked to reflect on their memories of their own grandmother and then share what they might find in their grandmother's trunk. Then everyone shares memories about their grand-parents. After everyone shares, the leader facilitates a discussion about their grandparent roles and how they think their grandchildren will remember them.

6. Life line of significant events: Participants are asked to draw a life line on a sheet of paper. On the line they note their birthdate and then list the significant events that they have experienced during their lifetime (e.g., World War II, Mexican Revolution, death of President Kennedy, first man to walk on the moon, invention of television, etc.). A discussion follows that encourages participants to share personal experiences around these events.

The group wraps-up with the leader's recognizing and supporting the sharing that occurred, and, if appropriate, asking participants to bring special item(s) for the next meeting. Written reminders, or having other staff help participants remember to bring objects, may be necessary.

Variations

Endless variations in focus activities. Similar format could be used with older children remembering when they were younger, and dealing with family changes.

Expected Outcome

A group experience in which participants shared personal feelings, and felt a common bond with others of the same age cluster. Participants also feel less isolated.

Special Strategies

As needed to respond to hearing, visual, or other participant limitations.

The Directive Group

Source

Kaplan, K., 1988. *Directive Group Therapy: Innovative Mental Health Treatment.* Thorofare, NJ: Slack, Inc.
See also:
Kaplan, K., 1986. The directive group: Short-term treatment for psychiatric patients with a minimal level of functioning. *American Journal of Occupational Therapy,* 40(7):474–481.

Description/Rationale

Patients with severe psychiatric problems or organic brain dysfunction are often confused, have problems with attention, and lack the social skills needed to profit from verbal psychotherapy. A reality-oriented group structure in which input and expectations fit with patient abilities can support the patient in the process of reorganization, and help decrease anxiety.

Group Goals

Patients will:

1. Participate in activities.
2. Interact with others around a task.
3. Attend group consistently.
4. Initiate activities within the group.

Selection Criteria

Persons with impaired ego organization, poor personal boundarying, impaired ability to initiate and carry through with activity (e.g., persons with severe depression, schizophrenic disorders, thought disorder, hyperactivity).

Group Structure

Size: six to twelve patients

Length of session: forty-five minutes, five times per week

Duration: two to three weeks

Environment

Short term, inpatient setting.

Stress on environmental boundaries, maintenance of safety, and the creation of a "playful" context.

Materials

Blackboard, a large clock.

Leader's Role (Co-leaders are suggested)

To structure meeting, to reinforce reality testing, to act as a role model.

Session Format

Each meeting is designed to be complete within itself.

Orientation: Review of group's name, the date, the group's purpose.

Introduction: Introduction of new members, review of member's names.

Warm-up Activities: Low-level demand, often designed to get participants physically mobile (ten to fifteen minutes).

Selected Focus Activity: Designed to be arousing, structured around patient's abilities to succeed (e.g., bean bag toss, magazine scavenger hunt, hangman, etc.) (twenty minutes).

Wrap-up: Reiterate what the group did during the session.

Expected Outcome

Patient is able to attend the group for forty-five minutes and receives a certificate of accomplishment at the end of the two to three week period.

Special Strategies

Kaplan suggests a post-group session in which staff critique the group activity session, while participants observe and listen to the critique.

Coronary Heart Disease and Daily Function

Source

Dell Orto, A.E. and R.G. Lasky, 1979. *Group Counseling and Physical Disability*. North Scituate, MA: Duxbury Press.

Description/Rationale

A structured group experience for patients who have coronary heart disease. The activity is designed to increase the patient's awareness of psychosocial changes that occur following a myocardial infarction (MCI) and the effect of these changes upon the patient's function in daily life.

Group Goals:

1. Patient will identify the changes in physical performance and their relationship to the patient's present psychosocial performance.
2. Patient will identify the changes that he or she experiences and the difficulties experienced when adapting to these changes.
3. Patient will identify the strategies for managing the changes and facilitating adaptation in daily life.

Selection Criteria

Persons and/or "significant others" of persons who have coronary disease.

Group Structure

Size: six to ten persons

Length of session: two hours

Duration: one-time or a part of a series of groups with a focus on a healthy life style or a support group

Environment

In- or outpatient setting, treatment of prevention focus.

Work surface for writing (table or clipboard).

Movable chairs for discussion circle and feedback sessions.

Materials

Paper and pencils, felt tip pen and flip chart or blackboard.

Leader's Role

Prepare worksheets.

Introduce group.

Distribute paper or worksheets and pencils.

Structure and monitor the activity.

Facilitate discussion and feedback.

Session Format

Introduction (summary about coronary disease, psychosocial aspects of cardiac disease, and purpose of the group).

Request participants to list the ways life has changed since MCI.

Request participants to note the difficulties they've experienced since these changes.

Use a round-robin approach and ask each group member to share the items listed.

Divide the group into pairs and ask the partners to brainstorm during a ten to fifteen minute period to identify ways to cope with the changes and the perceived difficulties.

Facilitate a large group discussion in which the members share the ideas that result from the brainstorming session.

Record the coping strategies on a flip chart for all the group members to see.

On a clean sheet of paper or form, ask each group member to list three changes that they wish to make and the strategies they could use to manage these changes, and facilitate copying with the changes needed to maximize function following a MCI.

Expected Outcome

Mutual support from peers who have had myocardial infarction and similar experiences. Participants practice problem-solving within the constraints of the disability and identify their capabilities for copying.

Special Strategies

None

Variations:

Begin the group with an activity which will help the participants identify recent changes or difficulties (e.g., a change checklist in which

Recent Changes	Difficulties	Coping Methods

Desired Changes: _____

_____

_____

Coping Strategies: _____

_____

_____

Figure 11.10a   Cardiac Function

items that relate to employment, daily routine, roles, and sexual activity [as well as others gleaned from cardiac research] are identified), or the "recent life changes survey" which identifies forty-two possible life changes in work, family, personal and interpersonal categories (p. 254 and 274. Group could be used for persons with any physical disability who are experiencing psychosocial changes that decrease functions in daily life. (See Figures 11.10a and 11.10b.)

Group Rehabilitation for Patients with Parkinson's Disease

Source

Gauthier, L., Danziel, S. and S. Gauthier, 1987. The benefits of group occupational therapy for patients with Parkinson's disease. *American Journal of Occupational Therapy* 41(6):360–365.

Recent Changes	Difficulties	Coping Methods
Fear of dying		?
Not want to be alone	Always want a family member with me	My family has adjusted their schedules and share time with me
Less energy	Go to bed by 9 PM or earlier	We watch TV together in bed.
Easily upset	Get angry with my family and tell them off	?

Desired Changes: 1. Be more pleasant (Therapist helps patient rephrase this to read, "Have more control over my feelings and how I express them.")

2. Increase my energy.

Coping Strategies: 1. I don't know

2. Do exercises daily to increase my energy level

Figure 11.10b Cardiac Function: Patient Example

Description/Rationale

Parkinson's disease is a degenerative disease which may cause limited physical function, depression and a feeling of social isolation. In addition to traditional physical rehabilitation approaches used, group treatment can provide a support group as well as an educational experience for learning about the disease process. The groups have been shown to be cost effective and to influence the participants' motivation, functional independence and interpersonal relationships.

Group Goals

1. Participants will maintain their mobility, dexterity, and ability to perform daily living skills.
2. Participants will gain a foundation of knowledge to understand the disease process.

3. Participants will establish a support/friendship network through social activities.

Selection Criteria

Patients with idiopathic Parkinson's disease. Patients in this study were ambulatory, lived at home, were willing to participate, and had bilateral involvement. (Note: We feel that this group format is a viable treatment approach for other persons who have chronic diseases such as arthritis.)

Group Structure

Size: eight people

Length of session: two-hour group, twice a week

Duration: five weeks

Environment

Outpatient, group rehabilitation program.

Leader's Role

Gives pre- and post-tests.

Introduces the group.

Leads exercises.

Structures and monitors the activities.

Facilitates discussion and feedback.

Session Format

Each group is divided into time periods which use functional activities, educational activities and informal socialization.

Group begins with socialization.

Warm-up exercises/mobility activities.

Rest and socialization.

Dexterity activities.

Functional activities.

Educational activities.

Informal socialization and group closure.

Activities

Activities use visual cues (modeling by therapist as well as mirrors in which patients can see themselves while exercising) and auditory cues (music and rhythm activities, singing and dancing) to facilitate balance, posture, walking, facial mobility, and range of motion.

Functional activities (games and crafts to maintain dexterity).

Educational activities (guest lectures, homework, literature on Parkinson's disease).

A therapy book can be provided which includes summaries of guest lectures, Parkinson literature, homework activities, and a section for personal notes.

Expected Outcome

Through controlled physical exercise, socialization and increased knowledge, the participants will maintain optimum physical function, have a sense of hope and improved quality of life, and will benefit from the support and friendships experienced in the group. In this study, patients maintained function during a one-year period. There was a decrease in bradykinesia and akathisia; patients reported greater sense of psychological well-being; patients had improved communication skills; and they had an increased understanding of Parkinson's disease.

Special Strategies

Sessions five through ten were videotaped. Patients were said to have benefited from viewing these tapes.

Family members were welcome to attend any of the treatment sessions.

Cognitive Group for Adults with Head Injury

Source

Lundgren, C. C. and E. L. Perschino, 1986. Cognitive Group: A Treatment Program for Head Injured Adults. *American Journal of Occupational Therapy*, 40(6):397–401.

Description/Rationale:

The therapists who created these groups felt that patients who have had a head injury can benefit from group treatment that would supplement the individual treatment programs in which the patients were participating. Group treatment was intended to provide an opportunity for the participants to identify with one another, to share common problems and achievements, and to develop competency in group skills through functional activities.

Group Goals

Both individual and group goals are described.

During the group participants will:

1. Develop problem solving strategies.
2. Improve memory (immediate recall and short-term memory).
3. Improve social skills.

Individual participant goals related to the following functional areas:

1. Improve organization, judgment, and reasoning skills.
2. Increase awareness of socially acceptable behavior.
3. Increase social interaction.
4. Improve self-image.
5. Decrease egocentricity.
6. Increase self-initiative.

Selection Criteria

Patients from fifteen to seventy-seven years of age have participated in the groups; 65 percent of the participants were fifteen to thirty-four years old. All were inpatients who had a traumatic head injury and functional problems (physical, emotional, social, perceptual, cognitive and communication/interpersonal). All had been and were presently involved in individual treatment; they had an awareness of their boundaries (of self and the environment), had improved in their orientation and attention, and had participated in a sensory stimulation group. Most were functioning at the Rancho Cognitive Function levels of V, VI, and VII.

Group Structure

Size: six patients

Length of session: thirty minutes, five times per week

Duration: patients participated from two to twenty-four weeks, the average was seven and one-half weeks

Environment

Inpatient setting, treatment focus.

A quiet, distraction free setting.

A controlled social environment.

Leader's Role

Plan activity groups for a one week period, record plan in the planning journal.

Introduce group.

Present, structure, and monitor the activity.

Facilitate discussion and feedback.

Record group outcome.

Session Format

Based upon a developmental frame of reference, three types of groups are used — parallel group, project group, and egocentric group. (Mosey 1969).

During parallel groups, the leader helps the participants complete the individual task they choose and responds to the social interactions that they initiate. Participants learn to attend to a task, and tolerate working in the same environment with others.

During the project group, the leader monitors the group activity and helps the participants complete the task within an identified time frame.

The leader of an egocentric cooperative group allows the participants to select, plan, and carry through with a long-term task. During the task, the leader facilitates socialization and cooperative work efforts as members try to satisfy their emotional needs. Completion of the task is secondary.

Activity

Structured and graded; tasks are varied, usually have some familiarity to the participants; may use simple to complex structures, and concrete to abstract reasoning.

Life skills training (map reading, locating community resources, ordering food from a menu).

Memory practice (games, reasoning and abstract stories, word scrambles).

Role play (emergency responses, responses to danger).

Expected Outcome

During each group experience, the participants will each experience success (usually achieved through the structure of the activity). Successes improve the participants' self-image, improve memory skills, and facilitate social interaction. Participants receive feedback regarding their social behavior.

Documentation

Participants' performance (behavior and social interaction) is evaluated bi-weekly by therapists who use an adapted version of the Occupational Therapy Functional Evaluation.

Special Strategies

The group, on Friday of each week, uses a cooking activity to promote working together and socialization. Therapists/leaders use this group as a "recap" of the week and to plan week-end activities.

Wheelchair Mobility Group

Source

Beresford, D., 1989. Model for a wheelchair mobility group. *Occupational Therapy Forum*, August 7.

Description/Rationale

The person who has had a cardiovascular accident and has a severe physical impairment has multiple needs, psycho-social as well as physical. During a group experience, these patients can satisfy some of their needs, learn and practice mobility skills, learn to cope with their disability, and make the transition back into the community.

Group Goals

1. Participants will share experiences with others who have similar disabilities and problems.
2. Participants will increase their physical endurance.
3. Participants will decrease their frustration with immobility.
4. Participants will increase their level of mobility independence.
5. Participants will gain skills for mobility independence in the community.

Selection Criteria

Persons who have had a CVA, having sitting balance (fair), neglect their hemiplegic side, have visual impairments, need assistance to propel wheelchair, have low endurance for activity, and coordination difficulties.

Group Structure

Open group in which there is a continuous flux of patients.

Size: not specified. Author's opinion: four to eight persons, depending upon the space available and the severity of functional problems.

Length of session: not specified. Author's opinion: twenty to sixty minutes, depending upon the endurance of the patients.

Duration: a series of groups in which four phases of skills are mastered: basic skills, technical ability, intermediate skills, and advanced skills.

Environment

Large open area that can accommodate the wheelchairs and the mobility exercises or the obstacle course route.

When patients are more skilled, areas throughout the hospital, hallways, outdoor patios, varied surfaces (smooth, grass, gravel etc.).

Community excursion to a local restaurant or to a shopping mall.

Materials

Educational materials that describe mobility problems, wheelchair care, and so on.

Written program at discharge.

Leader's Role

Assess the individual prior to the group.

Introduce the group.

Facilitate sharing of feelings, frustrations, successes, etc.

Provide instruction to increase understanding of one's disability (e.g., hemianopsia, etc.).

Introduce and monitor the activity, exercises, skill practice, obstacle course, community trips, automobile transfer, etc.

Session Format

Introduce the group and discuss its goals.

Give opportunity for participants to express frustrations.

Introduce the skills to be learned.

Pair patients with similar abilities.

Provide educational experiences: disability issues; wheelchair mechanics, parts, and accessories; and correct procedure for improving mobility.

Skill practice.

Encourage participants to help each other outside of the group (advise, praise, and instruct).

Variations

None listed.

Expected Outcome:

Participants had increased self-pride and confidence in their abilities to participate in the community. They were able to perform the necessary skills for mobility and more frequently went out into the community after they left the hospital.

Special Strategies

To increase the understanding of instructions by those persons with aphasia, the therapist uses the wheelchair and only one side of his or her body to demonstrate the mechanics and skills to be learned.

Drawing/Communication Group

Source

Oster, G. D. and P. Gould, 1987. *Using Drawings in Assessment and Therapy*. New York: Brunner/Mazel Publishers.

Description/Rationale:

Drawings (or other creative activities) are used as a catalyst for communication during group treatment. The drawings provide a concrete task which acts as a focus for member interactions. Drawings can promote the discussion of events that led to hospitalization and which are causing stress. They also can help clarify the participants' thoughts and feelings in their visual representation of personal images.

Group Goals

1. Patient will participate in a drawing activity and share personal reactions to the creative experience; participant shares at own comfort level.

2. Patient will increase personal awareness through the drawing experience and discussion.

3. Patient will assume responsibility for sharing art materials and returning them to storage.

Selection Criteria

Children through older adult ages who are oriented and boundaried and can benefit from increased personal awareness and communication activity groups.

Group Structure

Type: may be open or closed group

Size: not stated. Authors recommend eight to twelve persons depending upon the capabilities of the participants.

Length of session: seventy-five to one hundred minutes

Duration: one time, or one of a series of communication groups that use creative media

Environment

In- or outpatient setting.

Work surface for drawing or other creative activity.

Area that is private with few distractions to facilitate creative process and discussion.

Materials

Creative media — clay, paint, marking pens, color pencils, drawing paper, mural paper, collage materials.

Leader's Role

To provide a nonjudgmental climate and facilitate creative and spontaneous expression and interaction.

Structure the drawing group or creative experience as needed.

Identify the goals of the group.

Facilitate sharing among the group members.

Bring the group to a close by summarizing the experience and reiterating the goals and their relationship to functioning in the community.

Session Format

The leader introduces the group, the drawing activity, and its purpose.

During a half-hour period, the participants complete the drawing task. Suggestions: draw oneself, one's likes and dislikes, one's mask, oneself five years from now, what one wishes to change, one's feelings, oneself as others see one, a self-advertisement, objects of importance; shared drawings; or mural with a particular theme.

Leader facilitates a discussion about the drawing experience and the symbols that are represented. The leader helps the participants identify the personal meanings expressed and does not interpret the drawings nor their symbols.

Leader brings closure to the group.

Participants help the leader clean up and store all art materials.

Expected Outcome

A group experience which allows for verbal and nonverbal expression of thoughts and feelings and opportunity for increased self-awareness and communication with others.

Special Strategies

The therapist provides more structure for children's drawing/creative expression groups.

Older adults may hesitate to draw because they may see it as a "childish" activity. They are more likely to be interested in using oil or acrylic paints or marking pens. Avoid using crayons with older adults.

When participants resist drawing, the leader may offer them the opportunity to draw without having to share their drawings with others in the group.

When participants are "stuck" or unable to decide what to draw, the leader can encourage them to scribble and then look for images in their scribbles.

Variations

If patients have limited drawing ability, they may be able to make collages from magazine pictures or other available materials.

Endnotes

1. J. L. Moreno is identified as the originator of *psychodrama*, a therapeutic form that entails the intentional acting out of the various faces or roles of the individual as he or she interacts with others in their lives. Psychodrama may include the use of treatment staff or others as "auxiliary egos" who try to give expression to aspects of the person of which he or she is unaware.

   Sociodrama or *sociometric* techniques refer to the use of psychodrama methods within a group and towards the end of clarifying the personality and social structure of the group.

2. The term *therapeutic community* is attributed originally to Main in an article he published in 1946 entitled "The Hospital as a Therapeutic Institution". It is a concept popularized, however, by the work of Maxwell Jones in post-war Great Britain. In the late 1940s, Britain saw great numbers of physically and emotionally traumatized individuals returning from the war. The idea of a therapeutic community was, in part, a response to treat numbers of patients in excess of what could be handled by individual physicians. As described by Jones (1953) and as used today in health care, a therapeutic community is characterized by:

   1. A breakdown in the strict division between staff and patients.
   2. Patients being encouraged to bring their concerns to patient/staff community meetings to be resolved by the group, rather than by the traditional physician-as-authority.
   3. Patients involved in work, recreational, educational, and social experiences within the milieu.
   4. The group experience being viewed as a treatment agent.
   5. The milieu being viewed as a place for corrective learning experiences and for testing new skills (see Jones 1953).

3. Activity Group Therapy (AGT) was the name given to the treatment method developed by S. R. Slavson in the 1930s in New York City.

Slavson had a Freudian orientation to understanding objects and events, but in the design of AGT did not aim for uncovering unconscious material, rather at the improvement of interpersonal relationships. AGT was specifically for mid-age children who had relationship difficulties but were not severely disturbed; that is, they needed to have some level of ego and superego development before entering the group. Typically four to seven children were invited to attend a "club," in which they were to have fun, play games, and do activities. The aim was to allow children to take responsibility for the club's activities in an atmosphere that was highly permissive. It was assumed that without the interference of a "noxious" adult, the children would eventually take responsibility and work out healthy relationships among themselves. The adult-leader was to be "neutral" but sensitive and caring. The environment and its contents were carefully designed to be simple, not easily damaged by rough play, and without suggestive colors or materials. The group would last nine months to a year. While old in origin, the AGT model is still used in some groups (see MacLennan 1983; Slavson and Schiffer 1975).

4. The traditional analytically-oriented therapy group is a long-term group experience designed for adults with a functioning ego. The therapist-leader takes a neutral position (seldom divulging personal information), encouraging participants to project onto the therapist their own beliefs about a parent-figure, and to better understand and work through their feelings with the aid of timely therapist interpretation.

5. The *encounter group movement* flourished during the late 1960s and early 1970s. It grew up outside of the "establishment" — it is not typically associated with traditional medicine, university programs, or government grants. The *encounter group* is an intensive group experience (of usually eight to fifteen participants) that tends to emphasize personal growth and the development or improvement of interpersonal communication and relationships. In an encounter group the emphasis is on feedback, personal sharing in the here-and-now, openness, honesty, self-awareness and body awareness. Many non-traditional techniques have become associated with encounter including the "marathon" (lengthy meeting time), movement techniques, gestalt therapy techniques, massage, yoga, fantasy, and meditation. Directly involved with the advancement of encounter has been Esalen Institute in California (see Rogers 1970; Schutz; 1973).

6. Just because three people get together and have a good experience does not mean activity group therapy has occurred. In Group A, three individuals do share a task and most likely have a socially positive experience. But this is not an intentionally designed or monitored therapy experience as it is understood in a health care setting.

   We see Group B as a planned activity group, co-led by two staff members whose focus is on daily living skills. However, the exact nature of group goals are not specified, and whether or not this is a small group is not known.

   In our estimation, Group C is clearly a small therapeutic activity group, where patients come together for a well-defined purpose and where group interaction is used as a means to facilitate change.

7. *Cybernetics* is a term coined by engineer Norbert Weiner to describe the cycle in machines that enables them to be self-regulatory. The term literally means "self-steering." More broadly, cybernetics refers to computer technology, information theory, and self-regulating machines. Cybernetics represents a special case of general system theory.

8. As conceived by Abraham Maslow, human needs can be understood as existing in a hierarchy, with lower level or basic needs having to be satisfied before higher level needs can be addressed.

   Needs are those internal drives that impel human behavior. Usually presented as a pyramid (with basic needs at the bottom), human needs are classified into five main groups:

   Basic survival needs — the need for food, water, clothing.

   Safety needs — the need to be physically safe.

   Belongingness needs — the need to be affiliated with others.

   Ego-status needs — the need to feel effective and competent, and to have self-esteem.

   Self actualization needs — the need to reach one's potential; to be all one can be, and use one's special talents (see Maslow, 1970).

9. *Field theory* evolved from the movement known as "gestalt psychology" which originated in the early twentieth century with the work of such men as Wolfgang Kohler, Kurt Koffka, and Max Wertheimer. Kurt Lewin, also a gestalt psychologist, studied with these men in Germany following World War I. Lewin's field theory was an attempt to explain both personality and social behavior. It's chief premise is that behavior

is a function of the whole context or "field" that exists when the behavior occurs. Lewin believed that the person and the situation could be represented mathematically, and that positive and negative forces moving a person towards or away from an object or event could be graphically depicted in terms of the forces' direction (*vector*) and force (*valence*).

Lewin represented the person as having a permeable boundary and exiting within a psychological environment. The person plus their psychological environment he called the *life space*. The life space, he said, also had a permeable boundary and existed within the physical or outside world. Using the concept of a psychological reality, we can see that Lewin's theory was essentially phenomenological, as well as consistent with system theory (Hall and Lindzey, 1970). See endnote #12 for a discussion of a related concept, force field analysis.

10. Ecological theory draws from the work of Lewin (1931, 1935, 1951), Husserl (1950), Kohler (1938), Katz (1930), G. H. Mead (1934), Thomas and Thomas (1928), Sullivan (1947), Dewey (1913, 1916, 1931), Linton (1936), and Benedict (1934). It was developed and is used in systematic study of the interaction between individuals and their multilevel environment. The levels include: (1) the microsystem, or the person's immediate setting — the activity, role, and interpersonal relationships; (2) the mesosystem, or the multiple environments in which the person interacts — home, school, work, neighborhood; (3) the exosystem, the setting in which events occur that influence a person's life experience, but in which he or she does not directly interact — government and health care legislation, decision of the school board; and (4) the macosystem, or the culture and subculture — one's attitudes, beliefs, and ideologies. All of these systems interrelate and influence one's psychosocial growth, behavior, and changes that occur throughout life. The theory has been used in the development of psycho-social theories, in research and in clinical practice (see Bronfenbrenner, 1979).

11. There are several ways to look at the situation that exists when patients that have a variety of activities available are told to attend only the activities they wish. One idea is that if the therapist in charge of the activity plans a meaningful experience, patients will choose to attend and participate. Another belief is that having free choice allows patients to be responsible for themselves, and it better approximates the way they choose their own activities in daily life. A third consideration is that not every activity is necessarily beneficial to every

patient. Patients can be billed for just those activities that they feel are worthwhile and therefore attend.

12. *Force field analysis* was proposed by Kurt Lewin to identify the pressures or forces in an organizational system that either work towards or against change within the system.

Force can refer to any influence that facilitates the system, or that acts as an obstacle to change. The environment in which the system functions is referred to as the field; the forces can be viewed as *restraining forces* and *driving forces*. If desired changes are occurring, then driving forces are collectively stronger than restraining forces. If anticipated change is not occurring, then the reverse is true.

The forces acting for and against change can thus be labeled and analyzed. A change can then be facilitated by devising strategies to remove restraining forces and enhance supportive forces, or a combination (see Spier, 1973; Boshear and Albrecht, 1977).

Bibliography

Bachner, S., 1987. Group Process in a Community Occupational Therapy Cooking Group. In Ross, M., 1987, *Group Process*, Thorofare, NJ: Slack, Inc., p. 105–117.

Bales, R. F., 1955. The equilibrium problem in small groups. In Hare, A. P., Borgatta, E. F. and Bales R.F. (eds.), *Small Groups*. New York: Knopf.

Bales, R. F., 1950. *Interaction Process Analysis: A Method of Study of Small Groups*. Cambridge, MA: Addison-Wesley.

Bales, R. F., 1950. A set of categories for the analysis of small group interaction. *American Soc. Review,* 15:257–263.

Bammel, G. and Barrus-Bammel, L., 1982. *Leisure and Human Behavior.* Dubuque, IA: Wm. C. Brown Co.

Bandura, A., 1971. *Psychological Modeling: Conflicting Theories.* New York: Adine-Atherton.

Bandura, A., 1977. *Social Learning Theory.* Englewood Cliffs, NJ: Prentice-Hall, Inc.

Benne, K. D. and Sheats, P. 1948. Functional roles of group members. *Journal of Soc. Issues,* Vol. 4.

Bennis, W. and Shepard, H. 1956. A theory of group development. *Human Relations,* 9:415–437.

Bennis, W. and Shepard, H. 1961. Group observation. In Bennis, W., K. Benne, and R. Chin (eds.), *The Planning of Change.* New York: Holt, Rinehart and Winston.

Beresford, D., 1989. Model for a wheelchair mobility group. *Occupational Therapy Forum,* August 7, 1989.

Boshear, W. and Albrecht, K. 1977. *Understanding People: Models and Concepts.* La Jolla, CA: University Associates, Inc.

Brenner, P., 1984. *From Novice to Expert: Excellence and Power in Clinical Nursing Practice.* Reading, MA: Addison-Wesley.

Brilhart, J., 1978. *Effective Group Discussion* (3rd ed). Dubuque, IA: Wm. C. Brown Co.

Brill, N. P., 1985. *Working With People: The Helping Process* (3rd ed). New York: Longman.

Bronfenbrenner, U., 1979. *The Ecology of Human Development: Experiments by Nature and Design.* Cambridge, MA: Harvard University Press.

Bruce, M. and Borg, B. 1987. *Frames of Reference in Psychosocial Occupational Therapy.* Thorofare, NJ: Slack, Inc.

Bruner, J., 1966. *Toward a Theory of Instruction.* New York: W. W. Norton and Company.

Burnside, I. M. (ed.), 1978. *Working with the Elderly: Group Process and Techniques.* North Scituate, MA: Duxbury Press.

Butler, R. N., 1980–81. The life review: An unrecognized bonanza. *International Journal of Aging and Human Development,* 12(1):35–38.

Cartwright, D., 1951. Achieving change in people: Some applications of group dynamic thought. *Human Relations,* 4:381–392.

Cartwright, D., 1968. The nature of group cohesiveness. In Cartwright, D. and A. Zander (eds.). *Group Dynamics: Research and Theory.* New York: Harper and Row.

Clark, C., 1987. *The Nurse as Group Leader* (2nd ed.). New York: Springer Publishing Co.

Corey, L. N., 1978. Group techniques for effecting change in the more disturbed patient. *Group,* 2:149–160.

Corey, M. and Corey, G. 1987. *Groups: Process and Practice* (3rd ed.). Monterey, CA: Brooks/Cole Publishing.

Crootof, C., 1985. Poetry therapy for psychoneurotics. In Leedy, J. (ed.), *Poetry as Healer: Mending the Troubled Mind.* New York: The Vanguard Press.

Cutler, P., 1979. *Problem Solving in Clinical Medicine: From Data to Diagnosis.* New York: Basic Books, Inc.

Cynkin, S., 1979. *Occupational Therapy: Towards Health Through Activities.* Boston: Little, Brown and Company.

Dalley, T. (ed.), 1984. *Art as Therapy.* London and New York: Tavistock Publications.

deMaré, P. and Kreeger, L. 1974. *Introduction to Group Treatments in Psychiatry.* London: Butterworth and Co.

Dell Orto, A.E. and Lasky, R.G., 1979. *Group Counseling and Physical Disability.* North Scituate, MA: Duxbury Press, p. 381.

Dougherty, P. M. and Vining Radomski, M., 1987. *The Cognitive Rehabilitation Work Book.* Rockville, MD: Aspen Publications.

Doyle, P., 1986. Roles: Understanding Sources of Stress. In Pfeiffer and Goodstein (eds.). *The 1986 Annual: Developing Human Resources.* San Diego, CA: University Associates, p. 27–34.

Duncombe, L. and Howe, M., 1985. Group Work in Occupational Therapy: A Survey of Practice. *American Journal of Occupational Therapy,* 39(3):165.

Falk-Kessler, J. and Froschauer, M., 1978. The soap opera: A dynamic approach for psychiatric patients. *American Journal of Occupational Therapy,* 32(5):317–319.

Fidler, G., 1969. The task-oriented group as a context for treatment. *American Journal of Occupational Therapy,* 23:43–48.

Fisher, B. A., 1980. *Small Group Decision Making: Communication and the Group Process,* (2nd ed.). New York: McGraw-Hill Book Co.

Fluegelman, A. (ed.), 1976. *The New Games Book.* Garden City, NY: Doubleday and Co., Inc./Headlands Press.

Frank, J. D., 1957. Some determinants, manifestations and effects of cohesiveness in therapy groups. *International Journal of Group Psychotherapy,* 7:53–63.

Gauthier, L., Danziel, S., and Gauthier, S., 1987. The benefits of group occupational therapy for patients with Parkinson's disease. *American Journal of Occupational Therapy,* 41(6):360–365.

Glick, I., Clarkin, J., and Kessler, D., 1987. *Marital and Family Therapy* (3rd ed.) Orlande, Grune and Stratton/Harcourt Brace Jovanovich.

Greenberg-Edelstein, R., 1986. *The Nurturance Phenomenon: Roots of Group Psychotherapy.* Norwalk, CT: Appleton-Century-Crofts.

Gruen, W., 1979. Towards a theory of behavior changes in group therapy: A contemporary program of necessary inputs for the effective therapist. In Wolberg, L. and M. Aronson (eds.). *Group Therapy 1979: An Overview.* New York: Stratton Intercontinental Medical Book Corp.

Haffer, A., 1986. Facilitating change: Choosing the appropriate strategy. *Journal of Nursing Administration,* 16(4):18–22.

Hall, C. and Lindzey, G., 1970. *Theories of Personality* (2nd ed.). New York: John Wiley and Sons, Inc.

Hare, A. P., 1976. *Handbook of Small Group Research* (2nd ed.). New York: Free Press.

Hersey, P. and Blanchard, K., 1984. Situational leadership. In Tubbs, S., *A Systems Approach to Small Group Interaction* (2nd ed.). New York: Random House.

Heslin, R. and Dunphy, D., 1964. Three dimensions of member satisfaction in small groups. *Human Relations*, 17:99–112.

Hoffman, L., 1981. *Foundations of Family Therapy.* New York: Basic Books, Inc.

Homans, G. C., 1961. *Social Behavior: Its Elementary Form.* New York: Harcourt, Brace and World.

Howe, M., 1968. An occupational therapy activity group. *American Journal of Occupational Therapy*, 22(3):176–179.

Howe, M. and Schwartzberg, S., 1986. *A Functional Approach to Group Work in Occupational Therapy.* Philadelphia: J. B. Lippincott Co.

Ingersoll, B. and Goddman, L., 1980. History becomes alive. Facilitating reminiscence in a group of institutionalized elderly. *Journal of Gerontological Social Work*, 2(4):305–319.

Jones, M., 1953. *The Therapeutic Community: A New Treatment Method in Psychiatry.* New York: Basic Books, Inc.

Jones, J. E., 1980. Autographs: An Ice Breaker. In J. W. Pfeiffer and J. E. Jones, 1980. *The 1980 Annual Handbook for Group Facilitators* (9th annual). San Diego, CA: University Associates.

Kaplan, K., 1988. *Directive Group Therapy: Innovative Mental Health Treatment.* Thorofare, NJ: Slack, Inc.

Kaplan, K., 1986. The directive group: Short-term treatment for psychiatric patients with a minimal level of functioning. *American Journal of Occupational Therapy*, 40(7):474–481.

Kellerman, H. (ed.), 1981. *Group Cohesion: Theoretical and Clinical Perspectives.* New York: Grune and Stratton.

Knowles, M. and Knowles, H., 1959. *Introduction to Group Dynamics.* New York: Association Press.

Kramer, L., 1984. *SCORE: Solving Community Obstacles and Restoring Employment.* New York: Haworth Press.

Kwiatkowska, H. Y., 1978. *Family Therapy and Evaluation Through Art.* Springfield, IL: Charles C. Thomas Publisher.

Laben, J. and McLean, C., 1984. *Legal Issues and Guidelines: For Nurses Who Care for the Mentally Ill.* Thorofare, NJ: Slack, Inc.

Lakin, M., 1986. *Ethical Issues in the Psychotherapies.* New York: Oxford University Press.

Leopold, H., 1977. Selective group approaches with psychotic patients in hospital settings. *American Journal of Psychotherapy*, 30:95–105.

Lewin, K., 1951. *Field Theory in Social Science: Selected Theoretical Papers,* Cartwright, D. (ed.). New York: Harper and Row.

Liff, Z., 1979. A general systems approach to group leadership of borderline and narcissistic patients. In Wolfberg, L. and M. Aronson (eds.). *Group Therapy 1979: An Overview.* New York: Stratton International Medical Book Corp.

Lippit, G., 1973. *Visualizing Change: Model Building and the Change Process.* La Jolla, CA: University Associates.

Loomis, M., 1979. *Group Process for Nurses.* St. Louis: C. V. Mosby Co.

Lungren, C. C. and Perschino, E.L., 1986. Cognitive group: A treatment program for head injured adults. *American Journal of Occupational Therapy,* 40(6):397–401.

MacLennan, B., 1983. An activity group for preadolescent boys. In Rosenbaum, M. (ed.), 1983. *Handbook of Short-Term Groups.* New York: McGraw-Hill Book Co., p. 61–78.

Maslow, A. H., 1970. *Motivation and Personality* (2nd ed.). New York: Harper and Row.

Mattingly, C., 1988. Perspectives on clinical reasoning for occupational therapy. In Robertson, C. (ed.). *Mental Health Focus: Skills for Assessment and Treatment.* Rockville, MD: American Occupational Therapy Association.

May, P., Wexler, M.., Salkin J., and Schoop, T., 1978. Nonverbal techniques in the re-establishment of body image and self identity: A report. In Costonis, M. N. (ed.). *Therapy in Motion.* Urbana, IL: University of Illinois Press, p. 135–152.

Merritt, R. E. and D. D. Walley, 1977. *The Group Leader's Handbook: Resources, Techniques, and Survival Skills.* Champaign, IL: Research Press Co.

Miller, J. G. and Miller, D.D., 1981. Systems science: An emerging interdisciplinary field. *Center Magazine,* 14:44–55.

Morris, I. T. and Cinnamon,K.M., 1975. *A Handbook of Non-verbal Group Exercises.* Springfield, IL: Charles C. Thomas Publisher.

Mosey, A., 1981. *Occupational Therapy: Configuration of a Profession.* New York: Raven Press.

Mosey, A., 1973. *Activities Therapy.* New York: Raven Press.

Newel, A. and Simon, H., 1972. *Human Problem-Solving.* Englewood Cliffs, NJ: Prentice-Hall.

Nochajski, S. and Gordon, C., 1987. The use of Trivial Pursuit in teaching community living skills to adults with developmental disabilities. *American Journal of Occupational Therapy,* 41(1):10–15.

Oster, G. D. and Gould, P., 1987. *Using Drawings in Assessment and Therapy.* New York: Brunner/Mazel Publishers.

Pellagrino, E. and Thomasama, D., 1981. *A Philosophical Basis of Medical Practice.* New York: Oxford University Press.

Perry, D. and Bussey, K., 1984. *Social Development.* Englewood Cliffs, NJ: Prentice-Hall.

Rice, C. and Rutan, J., 1987. *Inpatient Group Psychotherapy: A Psychodynamic Perspective.* New York: Macmillan Publishing Co.

Rogers, C., 1970. *On Encounter Groups.* New York: Harper and Row.

Rose, S. D. and Jeffrey, L.E., 1987. *Working with Children and Adolescents in Groups.* San Francisco: Jossey Bass Publishers.

Ross, M. and Burdick, D., 1981. *Sensory Integration: A Training Manual for Therapists and Teachers for Regressed Psychiatric and Geriatric Patient Groups.* Thorofare, NJ: Slack, Inc.

Rubin, J. A. (ed.), 1987. *Approaches to Art Therapy.* New York: Brunner/Mazel Publishers.

Sampson, E. and Marthas, M., 1981. *Group Process for the Health Professions* (2nd ed.). New York: John Wiley and Sons.

Saretsky, T., 1977. *Active Techniques and Group Psychotherapy.* New York: Jason Aronson, Inc.

Schon, D., 1987. *Educating the Reflective Practitioner.* San Francisco: Jossey Bass Publishers.

Schon, D., 1983. *The Reflective Practitioner: How Professionals Think in Action.* New York: Basic Books, Inc.

Schutz, W., 1973. *Elements of Encounter: A Bodymind Approach.* Big Sur, CA: Joy Press.

Schutz, W., 1960. *FIRO: A Three-Dimensional Theory of Interpersonal Behavior.* New York: Rinehart-Wilson.

Schutz, W., 1971. *Here Comes Everybody.* New York: Harper and Row.

Schutz, W., 1967. *Joy.* New York: Grove Press.

Shaw, M., 1981. *Group Dynamics: The Psychology of Small Group Behavior* (3rd ed.). New York: McGraw-Hill.

Shaw, M., 1974. The Nature of Small Groups. In Cathcart, R. and L. Samover (eds.), 1974. *Small Group Communications: A Reader* (2nd ed.). Dubuque, IA: Wm. C. Brown Co.

Simon, H., 1972. *Human Problem Solving.* Englewood Cliffs, NJ: Prentice-Hall.

Slavson, S. R., 1950. *Analytic Group Psychotherapy with Children, Adolescents and Adults.* New York: Columbia University Press.

Slavson, S. R., 1961. Group psychotherapy and the nature of schizophrenia. *International Journal of Group Psychotherapy,* 11:3–32.

Slavson, S. R. and Schiffer, M., 1975. *Group Psychotherapies for Children: A Textbook.* New York: International Universities Press.

Smith, M., 1977. Conversion of Limitations. *Value Clarification.* CA: University Associates Publishers and Consultants.

Smith, M., 1977. Value Indicators: Time/Money. *Value Clarification.* La Jolla, CA: University Associates, Inc.

Spier, S., 1973. Kurt Lewin's force field analysis. In Jones, J. and J. Pfeiffer (eds.), 1973. *The 1973 Annual Handbook for Group Facilitators.* La Jolla, CA: University Associates.

Stanley, B. (ed.), 1985. *Geriatric Psychiatry: Clinical, Ethical and Legal Issues.* Washington, DC: American Psychiatric Press.

Stroud, M. and Sutton, E., 1988. *Activities Handbook and Instructor's Guide for Expanding Options for Older Adults with Developmental Disabilities.* Baltimore: Paul Brookes Publishing.

Sullivan, H. S., 1947. *Conceptions of Modern Psychiatry.* Washington, DC: W. M. Alanson White Psychiatric Foundation.

Thelen, H. and Dickerman, 1949. Stereotypes and growth of groups. In *Educational Leadership,* 6:309–316.

Tubbs, S., 1984. *A Systems Approach to Small Group Interaction.* New York: Random House.

Tuckman, B., 1965. Developmental sequence in small groups. *Psychological Bulletin,* 63:384–399.

Verny, T., 1974. *Inside Groups: A Practical Guide to Encounter Groups and Group Therapy.* New York: McGraw-Hill Book Co.

Von Bertalanffy, L., 1968. *General System Theory: Foundations, Development, Application* (rev. ed.). New York: George Braziller.

Walzlawick, P., J. Weakland and R. Fisch, 1974. *Change: Principles of Problem Formation and Problem Resolution.* New York: Norton.

Werner, H., 1948. *Comparative Psychology of Mental Development.* Chicago: Follett.

Werner, H., 1957. The conception of development from a comparative and organismic point of view. In Harris, D. (ed.), 1957. *The Concept of Development.* Minneapolis: University of Minnesota Press.

Woody, R., 1984. *The Law and the Practice of Human Services.* San Francisco: Jossey Bass Publishers.

Yalom, I., 1983. *Inpatient Group Psychotherapy.* New York: Basic Books, Inc.

Yalom, I., 1975. *The Theory and Practice of Group Psychotherapy* (2nd ed.). New York: Basic Books, Inc.

Index